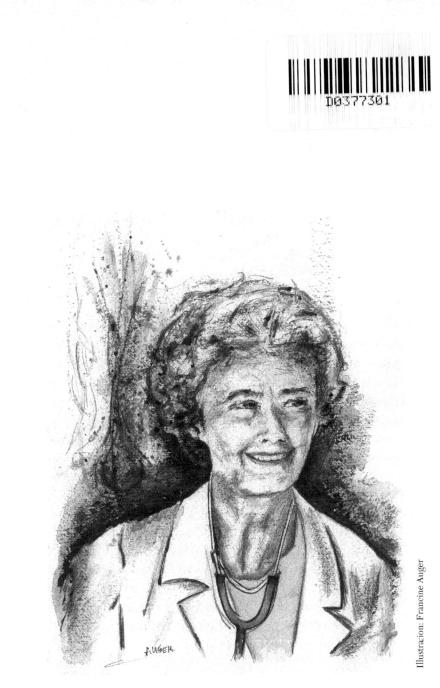

Lucille Teasdale, 1929-1996

Illustration: Francine Auger

Lucille Teasdale Corti C.M., M.D.

Deborah Cowley

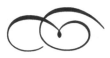

Deborah Cowley is an Ottawa-based writer and broadcaster. During her extensive worldwide travels, she has written over one hundred feature articles for different editions of *Reader's Digest* on such diverse subjects as chimpanzee guru Jane Goodall, the ORBIS flying eye doctors, and the pilgrim's path to Santiago de Compostela. She has worked on CBC television documentaries filmed in Egypt and prepared over fifty documentaries for CBC Radio. She has also written travel articles for various newspapers and travel magazines.

Deborah Cowley is the author of *Cairo, A Practical Guide* (University of Cairo Press), now in its twelfth edition. In the early 1990s, she collaborated with her husband George Cowley to write *One Woman's Journey: A Portrait of Pauline Vanier* (Novalis). Most recently, she edited the wartime letters of former Governor General Georges Vanier, published as *Georges Vanier: Soldier* (Dundurn Press).

In the same collection

Ven Begamudré, *Isaac Brock: Larger Than Life*.
Lynne Bowen, *Robert Dunsmuir: Laird of the Mines*.
Kate Braid, *Emily Carr: Rebel Artist*.
Kathryn Bridge, *Phyllis Munday: Mountaineer*.
William Chalmers, *George Mercer Dawson: Geologist, Scientist, Explorer*.
Gary Evans, *John Grierson: Trailblazer of Documentary Film*.
Judith Fitzgerald, *Marshall McLuhan: Wise Guy*.
lian goodall, *William Lyon Mackenzie King: Dreams and Shadows*.
Stephen Eaton Hume, *Frederick Banting: Hero, Healer, Artist*.
Naïm Kattan, *A.M. Klein: Poet and Prophet*.
Betty Keller, *Pauline Johnson: First Aboriginal Voice of Canada*.
Michelle Labrèche-Larouche, *Emma Albani: International Star*.
Wayne Larsen, *A.Y. Jackson: A Love for the Land*.
Francine Legaré, *Samuel de Champlain: Father of New France*.
Margaret Macpherson, *Nellie McClung: Voice for the Voiceless*.
Dave Margoshes, *Tommy Douglas: Building the New Society*.
Marguerite Paulin, *René Lévesque: Charismatic Leader*.
Raymond Plante, *Jacques Plante: Behind the Mask*.
T.F. Rigelhof, *George Grant: Redefining Canada*.
Arthur Slade, *John Diefenbaker: An Appointment with Destiny*.
Roderick Stewart, *Wilfrid Laurier: A Pledge for Canada*.
John Wilson, *John Franklin: Traveller on Undiscovered Seas*.
John Wilson, *Norman Bethune: A Life of Passionate Conviction*.
Rachel Wyatt, *Agnes Macphail: Champion of the Underdog*.

Lucille Teasdale

Library and Archives Canada Cataloguing in Publication
Cowley, Deborah, 1937-

    Lucille Teasdale: doctor of courage

    (The Quest library; 25)
    Includes bibliographical references and index.
    ISBN 1-894852-16-8

    1. Teasdale, Lucille. 2. Surgeons – Québec (Province) - Biography. 3. Surgeons – Africa – Biography. I. Title. II. Series: Quest library; 25.
RD27.35.T42C68 2005   617′.092   C2005-940770-0

Legal Deposit: Second quarter 2005
Library and Archives Canada
Bibliothèque nationale du Québec

XYZ Publishing acknowledges the support of The Quest Library project by the Book Publishing Industry Development Program (BPIDP) of the Department of Canadian Heritage. The opinions expressed do not necessarily reflect the views of the Government of Canada.

The publishers further acknowledge the financial support our publishing program receives from The Canada Council for the Arts, the ministère de la Culture et des Communications du Québec, and the Société de développement des entreprises culturelles.

Chronology: Valerie Firth
Index: Darcy Dunton
Layout: Édiscript enr.
Cover design: Zirval Design
Cover illustration: Francine Auger
Photo research: Deborah Cowley and Dominique Corti
Photos used by permission of Dominique Corti and the Lucille Teasdale and Piero Corti Foundation, www.lacorhospital.org

Printed and bound in Canada

XYZ Publishing
1781 Saint Hubert Street
Montreal, Quebec H2L 3Z1
Tel: (514) 525-2170
Fax: (514) 525-7537
E-mail: info@xyzedit.qc.ca
Web site: www.xyzedit.qc.ca
International Rights: Contact André Vanasse, tel. (514) 525-2170 # 25

Distributed by: Fitzhenry & Whiteside
195 Allstate Parkway
Markham, ON L3R 4T8
Customer Service, tel: (905) 477-9700
Toll free ordering, tel: 1-800-387-9776
Fax: 1-800-260-9777
E-mail: bookinfo@fitzhenry.ca

E-mail: andre.vanasse@xyzedit.qc.ca

DEBORAH COWLEY

TEASDALE

Lucille

THE QUEST LIBRARY

DOCTOR OF COURAGE

XYZ
Publishing

In grateful memory of

Dr. Lucille Teasdale
Dr. Piero Corti
Dr. Matthew Lukwiya

who devoted their lives to others

Contents

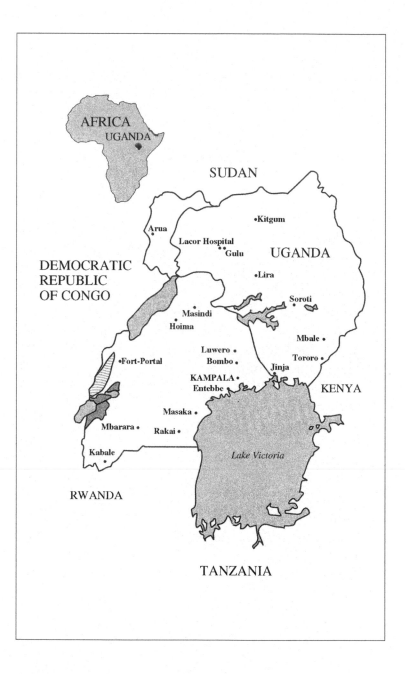

Preface

In October 1989 I had the good fortune to visit Lucille Teasdale and her husband, Piero Corti, in northern Uganda. Lucille had received an award from the Canadian Medical Association, and the *Reader's Digest* had asked me to investigate whether or not she would make a good subject for an article. I quickly discovered that, apart from this award, Lucille was virtually unknown in her native Canada. Few people knew her name and little had been written about her. Furthermore, the Canadian High Commission in Kenya was only vaguely aware of her presence in neighbouring Uganda, and none of their staff had ever met her or visited her.

From the little information I could find, I sensed that Lucille Teasdale was a woman who was out of the ordinary. After all, she had left her home in Montreal twenty-eight years earlier and travelled to the distant country of Uganda. There, she had lived and worked through long periods of horrendous political upheaval but had never succumbed to the temptation of returning to the safety of Canada. In 1987, I decided to write to Lucille and ask if I could visit her when I was next in East Africa.

Lucille replied at once. She was more than happy to help, she said, but with Uganda still in the midst of political turmoil, she felt it was much too dangerous for me to visit.

I wrote to Lucille the next year, but still she feared for my safety. Another year later, I was planning a trip to East Africa and asked again if I could include a visit with her in Uganda. Finally she agreed, but only if I would meet her and her doctor husband Piero Corti in Kampala and travel the eight-hour journey north to Lacor Hospital with them in the security of their Red Cross ambulance.

At long last, we managed to meet in Kampala. I was immediately struck by the strength of this woman. She was slight in build but expansive in spirit, and her bubbly personality quickly put me at ease.

We climbed into the front seat of the vehicle and Piero took the wheel. Throughout the journey, Lucille talked at fever pitch. She spoke in a heavily accented English, lacing her words with French and Italian expressions, her hands gesticulating for emphasis. As we bounced along, lurching to avoid the endless string of potholes, she seemed oblivious to the crumbling roadway or to the soldiers who stopped us regularly at gunpoint to check through the boxes of medical supplies in the van.

At sundown, we veered west of the northern town of Gulu. As we approached the hospital, the gates swung open and pandemonium broke out. A large group of nurses suddenly burst into a rhythmic song of welcome, and hordes of youngsters swarmed around the van in a heartfelt outpouring of affection for the couple they called "our beloved doctors."

During the week I spent with Lucille, I followed her on her daily hospital rounds while she checked on the progress of dozens of patients. I stood perched at her elbow while she undertook the most delicate operations, and I chatted with her long into the night about the frustrations and joys of her life in Uganda. I left at the end of the week much enriched and knowing I had met a truly remarkable woman, one of selfless dedication and immense courage.

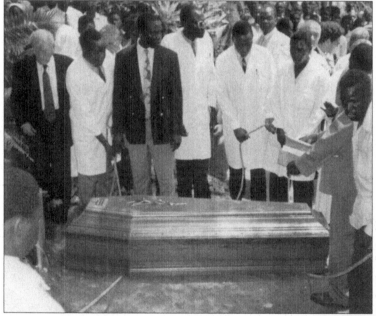

The coffin of Lucille Teasdale is lowered into the ground
by Medical Superintendent Dr. Matthew Lukwiya and a team
of doctors who are among the many trained by "Dr. Lucille."

1

A Sad Farewell

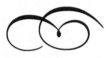

Lucille Teasdale was nothing less than a miracle worker... By her very presence, she gave Ugandans so much hope.
– Dr. Elizabeth Hillman, Canadian pediatrician

On a hot and steamy morning in August 1996 a small Cessna airplane landed on the airstrip of Gulu airport in northern Uganda. The door opened, and Piero Corti, an Italian doctor, stepped down onto the sizzling tarmac. Following close behind him was the coffin of his Canadian-born wife, Dr. Lucille Teasdale.

The moment ended an emotional journey for Corti, one he had dreaded ever since he first received news of Lucille's illness just over eleven years before. Since then, the two had lived through many highs and lows, and even as Lucille grew slowly weaker, they had both prayed for more time together. But it was not to be. After a heroic struggle that amazed her family and friends, Lucille finally lost the battle. Her death in Italy ended a remarkable and loving partnership that spanned thirty-five years and three continents.

On this blistering day, Corti was bringing his wife's body back to the country they had both called home for more than three decades. From the Gulu airport, a van carried the coffin across the barren plains of Uganda's northern region to the village of Lacor [pronounced *La-chore*]. After a bumpy six-kilometre journey, they arrived at a grove of palm trees. Branches of scarlet bougainvillea tumbled over a high stone wall, and a white sign with a large red cross marked the entrance to Lacor Hospital.

The van passed through the black steel gates and entered the compound. In front of them lay the hospital that was Piero and Lucille's lifelong labour of love. In 1961, when they first arrived here, they had found a tiny forty-bed dispensary run by a handful of Italian nuns. By 1996, they had managed to transform it "by our wits and our faith" into the medical showpiece of Uganda, a hospital with 450 beds and a staff of 400, all of them African.

Piero Corti had the coffin placed in the tiny hospital chapel. The following day, mourners began to arrive from all over the region. Some travelled by bus or bicycle but most came on foot. They lined up patiently in the hospital courtyard, then filed slowly through the chapel to pay their final respects to the person they called "Dr. Lucille," their surgeon and friend, who had cared for so many of them.

Over the years, Lucille Teasdale had given much to the people of her adopted country. She had restored the health of those she could. To those she could not cure, like the thousands who suffered from AIDS, she offered sympathy and comfort. Lucille was only too aware of the ravages of the human immunodeficiency virus (HIV). She was one of its victims.

A religious ceremony was held in the Cathedral in nearby Gulu, and local dignitaries came to pay homage and to offer prayers and tributes. Then the body was returned to the hospital compound for burial. Lucille had chosen the exact spot where she wished to be buried: she wanted to lie within sight of the hospital "so I can keep an eye on things." She also wished to be close to the tiny chapel where she and Piero had been married thirty-five years earlier.

Dr. Matthew Lukwiya, the hospital's senior medical advisor, stood solemnly beside the coffin. Six other Ugandan doctors, all wearing their white medical coats, lined up beside him. They were among the hundreds of Africans who had been trained by Lucille. Together, they lifted the coffin and slowly lowered it into the ground next to a flowering frangipani tree.

Piero Corti stepped slowly forward and placed a wreath of red roses on his wife's grave. A young African woman placed another wreath with a message tacked to it that read: "From a representative of the patients." She had been the last person to be treated by Dr. Lucille.

As a final tribute, each person stepped forward and tossed a flower into the grave before it was covered with earth.

Then the local Acholi people offered their final farewell. They did so in the form of their traditional funeral dance, one normally reserved for a tribal chief.

A dozen dancers moved forward. They carried spears and shields and wore headdresses of ostrich plumes and garments made of leopard skins. The dancers formed a circle around a band of drummers. The lead drummer signalled the start of the ceremony with a loud drum roll. Then a young man launched into a frenetic dance to the clatter of jingling hand-bells. The drumbeat continued.

A group of women shuffled into the circle in single file. They moved slowly and rhythmically, their bodies pumping to the beat of the drums. They sang and ululated in shrill piercing wails. One carried a framed portrait of Lucille, while the rest waved palm branches. Many dabbed tears from their eyes. The throbbing drumbeat rolled on.

Lucille Teasdale had touched the lives of many people. She may have left them, but clearly she would not soon be forgotten.

2

A Doctor in the Making

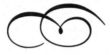

Everyone tried to discourage me from choosing surgery… They told me it was clearly a man's world and that no mother would ever put her child's life in the hands of a woman surgeon.
— Lucille Teasdale, 1956

Lucille Teasdale was born on 30 January 1929, the fourth in a family of five girls and two boys. They lived in Guybourg, a working-class neighbourhood in the east end of Montreal, where Lucille's father, René, a butcher, owned and ran the first grocery store in the area. Actively involved in the community and in his Catholic church, he left Lucille's mother, Juliette, with the job of raising their seven children.

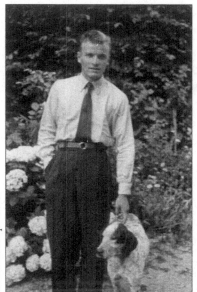

Piero Corti, a young Italian doctor, comes to Montreal to study pediatrics.

Lucille obtains her medical diploma *cum laude* at the Université de Montréal in 1955.

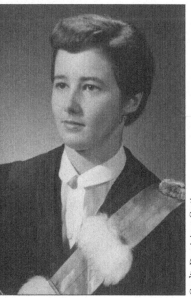

Lucille preferred skating and playing hockey on a nearby rink to helping at home with household chores. Having such a boisterous tomboy for a daughter annoyed Juliette, who was obsessed with neatness and cleanliness and thought that all young girls should be obedient and feminine.

Lucille's mother was a fragile woman who did her best to bring up her children according to her values. For most of her life, however, Juliette was given to long periods of depression. Lucille often noticed that her mother rarely smiled and always looked unhappy, but she was too young to understand why. Then one day, when Lucille returned from school, she overheard her mother confiding in a friend about her sadness. She had been so happy with her first three children, who were all girls, Juliette explained to her friend. But she desperately wanted a boy. When she was pregnant again, she prayed for a boy, but to her great disappointment, her fourth child was another girl. Lucille winced as she quickly realized she was that girl and the cause of her mother's unhappiness. She was devastated. From then on, she felt rejected by her mother, and the feeling haunted her for years.

Unlike her family and friends, Lucille loved school and worked hard at her studies. "None of them ever thought of studying," she recalled years later. "They all wanted to leave school as soon as possible. The boys wanted to work in a factory and the girls wanted to work in Macdonald's Tobacco."

Lucille was twelve when her parents sent her to a strict convent high school in Montreal. One day, a group of missionary nuns visited the school. They had just returned from China, and they talked about their work in an orphanage looking after Chinese babies. Lucille was fascinated by the stories of their work. That very day she decided, "I want to help poor and needy children. I'm going to do that by becoming a doctor!"

The only person she told was her father. "A doctor?" he said. "Yes," Lucille replied with certainty. "And I want to work in India." Her father was stunned. None of his other children showed any interest even in finishing high school, and Lucille was talking about a career that would require many long years of study.

He was also aware that Montreal in the 1950s, like most of the province of Quebec, was a very conservative society. Career opportunities were limited, especially for women. Many chose to be nurses or teachers and some became nuns. He pointed out that it was almost unheard of for a woman to train as a doctor, a career traditionally reserved for men.

But Lucille was not deterred. "I want to be a doctor, so I will just have to find a way."

Her father was clearly proud that she wished to continue her studies and did everything he could to help her. With his support, she studied even harder at school, managed to score top marks in her final examinations, and was awarded a bursary to attend Collège Jésus-Marie, one of the most prestigious classical colleges for women in Montreal, where she would complete high school. She was the only one in her family to do so.

At the college, Lucille met Dr. Jeanne Marcelle Dussault, a well-known woman doctor from Montreal who came to speak to the students. Lucille had already read about Dr. Dussault and was inspired by her example. *Here is a woman, a French Canadian and a doctor,* she thought. Having Dr. Dussault as a role model increased her determination to reach her goal.

With her mind fixed firmly on a medical career, Lucille continued to be a dedicated student. After four years at the college, she won a scholarship to enter the school of medicine at the Université de Montréal. She was twenty-one.

∽

The day in September 1950 when Lucille first walked into the Université de Montréal's medical school, she knew she was entering a man's world. Still, she was astonished to discover that, in her class of 110 students, there were only eight women. Her father had been right, but even he was surprised. "Only eight?" he asked, incredulously.

"Yes, and this is a big year for women!" Lucille laughed.

Lucille was a keen and bright student. She was also strikingly attractive, tall and slender with wavy blonde hair and big brown eyes. In spite of her inferiority complex – she always thought others were better and brighter than she was – she was popular with her first year classmates, who elected her Miss Medicine. Others too noticed this bright young student: when the Quebec publication *Le Petit Journal* was looking for a university student to feature on its cover for the October 1951 edition, they chose a photo of the budding doctor Lucille Teasdale giving an injection to a rabbit!

In 1955, Lucille graduated from medical school *cum laude*. She had decided to specialize in surgery and began her internship at Ste-Justine's children's hospital in Montreal. She was the only woman in her class to choose surgery. She thought women were made for surgery, that it was women's work – like sewing.

Few were convinced. All her friends tried to discourage her from choosing surgery. "Surgery is a man's world," one of them told her. Another took her aside and gave her an even stronger warning: "No mother would ever put her child's life in the hands of a woman surgeon," she said.

Lucille was determined to silence the sceptics. She would show her male colleagues that she was as good as they were. So she worked twice as hard, often for sixteen hours a day, seven days a week. Finally, after five gruelling years, she successfully completed her training and became one of Quebec's first female surgeons.

∽

Lucille was working at Ste-Justine's when a friend introduced her to a young Italian doctor who had come to Montreal to study pediatrics. His name was Piero Corti. She took little notice of him at first, but he later approached her in the hospital corridor and reintroduced himself. Piero was a good-looking young man, short and stocky, with a sparkle in his eyes and an engaging smile. She found him charming and amusing to be with, and she couldn't stop laughing at the way he spoke both French and English with a singsong Italian accent. But Lucille was so engrossed in her studies that she did not give him another thought. Piero, however, was immediately attracted by the beauty and intensity of this young intern.

The two came from very different backgrounds. Lucille had grown up in a working-class district of Montreal, while Piero was the son of a wealthy textile manufacturer from Milan, the fifth in a family of ten. At school, Lucille strove to excel, but Piero preferred sports and fast motorbikes to homework. Despite their comfortable circumstances, Piero's parents encouraged all their children to follow a profession, so he chose medicine and obtained a medical degree. He studied radiology and anesthesiology at the University of Milan.

Like Lucille, Piero was attracted by the idea of living and working in the Third World. One of his brothers was a Jesuit missionary in Chad, West Africa. A brother-in-law had served as a doctor, first in India and then in Africa. Their stories fascinated him and he was determined to follow in their footsteps.

Lucille had still to complete the final stage of her training. In order to practise as a surgeon, she needed one further diploma that required a period of training to be taken outside Canada. She sent letters to twenty top hospitals in the United States asking to be admitted to their surgical residence program. All twenty turned her down.

Lucille was absolutely furious. *I have an excellent academic record and impressive credentials. It must be the fact I'm a woman that has ruined my chance of a job in the United States*, she realized. She buried her anger and decided instead to apply for a job in France. She immediately received offers of positions in both Paris and Marseilles.

She chose Marseilles, a bustling Mediterranean seaport in the south of France. Now thirty-one years old, she said goodbye to her friends and family, and in September 1960, her father drove her to New York, where she boarded the S.S. *Liberté*.

After a five-day crossing, they reached the French port of Le Havre. Lucille boarded the train for the journey south. She grew increasingly excited as they flew past charming French villages with red-tiled roofs. As they moved south, she could feel the heat of the sun and marvelled at the luminescence of the countryside that so captivated Impressionist painters such as Van Gogh and Cézanne.

She caught her first sight of the Mediterranean when she reached Marseilles, a noisy and crowded city bordering the sea. She moved in with a French family and started work at once as an intern in pediatric surgery at the Hôpital de la Conception.

Lucille adjusted quickly to life in Marseilles. She made many new friends, but she was startled by their ignorance of Canada. "In Montreal, do you have snow ten months a year?" one of them asked. "Is there ever any sun? What language do you speak?" inquired another. They were very surprised when she told them that many Canadians living in Montreal speak French at school, at university, even in the shops. They were just as surprised when she told them that in summer, Montrealers grow tomatoes! They thought Montreal must always be much too cold.

She was amused to discover that the French spoken in France was different from the French she had learned in Canada. "The people here have difficulty understanding me because we have such different accents and different expressions," she told her sister Lise. "Here, the children always call me 'madam.' At the hospital, the nurses call me 'mademoiselle,' the interns and several doctors call me 'miss,' and the boss, when he needs me, says 'Go and find my Canadian.'"

∽

Lucille's plan was to spend eight months in Marseilles before heading to Paris to finish her internship there. She was so caught up in her new life that she thought little about the Italian doctor she had met at Ste-Justine's. Meanwhile Piero had left Montreal to work first with his brother in Africa and later with a friend who ran a hospital in India. During his travels, Piero had thought often about his meeting with Lucille in Montreal, and they had exchanged a few letters. Now that he was back home in Italy, he decided to visit her in Marseilles.

One day, Lucille arrived home from the hospital and was surprised to find Piero waiting on her doorstep. "What are you doing *here*?" she asked. He looked a little sheepish as he explained: "You see, I have been thinking about you so often that I decided I would come and tell you all about my travels."

He invited her for dinner in the Old Port of Marseilles. They chose a table by the water's edge where they could hear the sea lapping against the breakwater. Piero ordered bouillabaisse, the hearty fish soup that is a popular specialty of the region, and a bottle of wine. As they savoured the meal, he talked about his trip.

He had visited many different medical projects in Africa, both in Chad and in the Congo. He had also worked for a period in India. But it was during a visit to Uganda that he had made an exciting discovery. "A friend took me to the north of the country to see a small dispensary, St. Mary's Hospital, near the village of Lacor," he explained. "The clinic is tucked away in a remote corner of the region and has just forty beds. It is run by a dozen Italian missionary nuns, the Comboni sisters, who serve as nurses and midwives." He paused, sipped some wine, and continued. "The minute I saw the facility, I knew this could be the answer to my dream to build a world-class hospital in a Third World country."

Piero was also deeply moved by the beauty of Uganda, a country that was eagerly approaching its independence from Britain in 1962. He described his impressions to Lucille and talked about his plans to build a hospital that would provide specialized services to supplement those of the district hospital in nearby Gulu. "My fondest dream," Piero added, wide-eyed with excitement, "is that, in time, this small hospital could become one of the best in Uganda and one that would be completely run by Africans."

As he talked about his plans, Piero spoke faster and faster. "I know that what I am talking about is a gigantic task, but I feel certain that, with God's help, I can make it happen." On the more practical side, he believed that he could handle all the administrative duties of the new facility. He could recruit doctors from Italy and train nurses locally. "But most important of all," he added, "I need someone with experience in surgery."

There was a long, silent pause as Piero braced himself to pose the question: "Lucille, why don't you come to Uganda and help out in the hospital for two or three months?"

Lucille was stunned. She hardly knew Piero and she knew almost nothing about Uganda. As the meal progressed, Piero's childlike enthusiasm became infectious. "I will even offer to pay your airfare plus money for cigarettes and toothpaste," he said.

Lucille laughed. "You are very, very persistent."

Piero left for Milan and Lucille pondered the idea of joining him in Africa. She was enjoying her life in Marseilles and was anxious to complete her course. But she found herself thinking more and more about Piero's offer. Here was the chance to live out her childhood ambition to be a doctor in the Third World. She suddenly found herself thinking, *Why not?*

∽

As Christmas approached, Piero telephoned her from Milan and asked her to join his family for the festive season. Lucille saw this as a good chance to get to know him better before making a final decision. She was also curious to meet his family. He had spoken of them often and appeared to enjoy an especially close relationship with his parents, something she had lacked in her own childhood. Just before Christmas, she boarded the train for Milan.

Piero met her at the railway station and they travelled together to Besana in Brianza, the town where his parents lived, an hour's drive from Milan. As they approached the family home, she couldn't believe her eyes: their house was a huge mansion standing on vast grounds ringed with palm trees. The interior was even more lavish, with large family portraits lining the walls and maids in frilly white aprons floating from room to room.

Piero's family welcomed her warmly, curious about this new arrival. In her presence, they all spoke to her in French or English, then among themselves switched effortlessly into Italian. Though they could not have been more welcoming, Lucille couldn't stop thinking about her own modest upbringing in the east end of Montreal, and she felt uncomfortable and out of place.

The next night, Piero took her to a performance of the ballet *Cinderella* at La Scala, the world-famous opera house in Milan. She was overwhelmed by the opulence of the auditorium, its five semicircular tiers of boxes reaching upwards to the ornate ceiling. They sat, as if in a dream, watching the fairy-tale story unfold. At intermission, as Piero poured a glass of champagne, Lucille cast aside any misgivings and told him: "Yes, I will join you in Uganda. But I must make it clear that it is only for a month or two." They raised their glasses in a toast to the future.

Lucille returned to Marseilles and prepared to leave for Africa.

3

Baptism by Fire

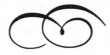

I always thought that all of Africa was a jungle, so imagine my surprise to find a forty-bed hospital virtually in the middle of nowhere. For a population of 40,000, I am the only surgeon able to do certain operations. Fortunately, I brought along my surgery textbooks.
— Lucille Teasdale, 3 May 1961

On 2 May 1961, Lucille joined Piero in Milan and together they boarded a UN military plane that would take them to Uganda. As it lifted off, Lucille was bursting with excitement. This was her first trip to Africa and the beginning of a thrilling new adventure.

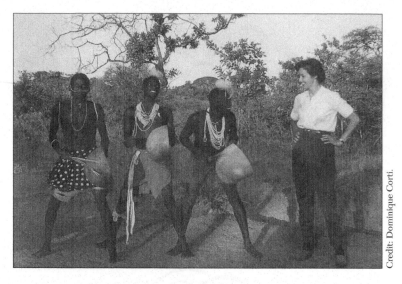

Acholi drummers give Lucille a noisy African welcome
on her arrival in May 1961.

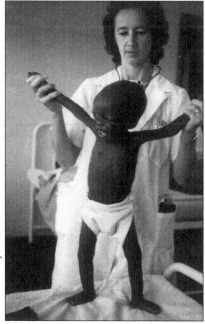

Dr. Lucille checking over a
new admission.

They flew slowly southward, and she watched with fascination as they crossed the blue expanse of the Mediterranean. Then she spotted its southern shoreline and knew this must be Egypt. The arid desert stretched as far as she could see, while the Nile River threaded its way south into the heart of Africa until it reached Uganda, where it emptied into one of the largest lakes in Africa, Lake Victoria.

Uganda is a relatively small country, about the size of Newfoundland, and completely landlocked. It is, however, blessed with an abundance of lakes and rivers, a rich and fertile soil, and a string of national parks.

The couple landed at Entebbe, Uganda's principal airport, which is perched on the edge of Lake Victoria just thirty-five kilometres west of the capital, Kampala. Looking across the lake, Lucille could see the distant peaks of the Ruwenzori Mountains, more often known as the Mountains of the Moon. Uganda was just as Piero had described it – a land of the most breathtaking beauty.

On the airport tarmac, the Union Jack flapped in the breeze and reminded visitors that the country had for many years been a colony of Britain. But the next year, in October 1962, the colony would gain its independence and the people of Uganda would finally run their own country. The excitement was palpable.

Brother Toni Biasin, one of the Italian Comboni missionaries, known as the Verona Fathers, met Lucille and Piero at the airport and drove them into Kampala. They found it to be a dynamic modern city, built, like Rome, on seven hills. There were handsome shops and large banks, an abundance of restaurants and cafés and huge stately mansions. Flowering trees and brilliant red poinsettia shrubs lined the wide avenues, and street vendors manned stalls laden with pyramids of fresh fruit – mangoes and pineapples, grapefruits and papayas.

The couple spent their first night in Kampala, and early the next morning, Brother Toni packed them into his old Peugeot and they set out for the long drive north. On the outskirts of town, Lucille spotted the signs of poverty that would become all-too-familiar: long stretches of flimsy shacks housing large extended families all jammed together under one shaky roof. Never before had she seen people living in such basic conditions.

The three-hundred-kilometre journey north would take them most of the day. Along the way, they passed hectares of deep green banana trees and huge coffee plantations that stretched as far as the eye could see. On the roadside, women in long multicoloured robes walked with babies slung on their backs in a hammock-like shawl. Some balanced giant water jugs on their heads while schoolchildren skipped along beside them, their bulging schoolbags strapped to their backs.

The farther north they travelled, the more barren the land became, eventually turning into rolling savannah – parched grasslands dotted with skeletal trees. Soon, they began to see tiny round huts with thatched beehive domes planted among fields of bamboo and eucalyptus. This was the land of the Acholi, the people they had come to serve.

∞

It was dusk when Lucille and Piero finally reached Gulu, a town of 40,000 people. Here, they turned off the main road and drove another ten kilometres until they saw the small sign to St. Mary's Hospital. "I have never felt so far from civilization," Lucille said. "It seems strange to have a hospital in such a remote corner of the land."

They passed through the gate and into the compound where three Acholi drummers beat out a noisy welcome. Sister Anna Pia, one of the team of Italian Comboni missionary nuns who ran the dispensary, stepped forward to greet them. She took Lucille by the arm and showed her to their residence, a small building with a wraparound veranda. "This is where you will be staying," she told Lucille. Piero would sleep in another building.

Before nightfall, Sister Anna Pia gave them a tour of the facility. The "hospital" consisted of one small building with only forty beds. Four nuns, a nurse, and a midwife ran the outpatient clinic, and a maternity unit housed half a dozen newborn infants.

That first night, as she was unpacking her bags, Lucille's head was spinning with excitement. Before she went to bed, she sat down and wrote to her sisters: "I always thought that all of Africa was a jungle so I was very surprised to find a forty-bed hospital at St. Mary's mission. For a population of 40,000, I am practically the only surgeon able to do certain operations. Fortunately, I brought all my surgery textbooks. It is very stressful but at the same time it is fascinating because I have the possibility of doing so much for these people."

The next morning, as Lucille walked over to the clinic, she passed a long line of patients who stood silently waiting for treatment. She set to work right away. She started off by visiting a small ward with twice as many patients as beds and began her examination rounds, carefully checking each person in turn. Suddenly, Sister Anna rushed in. "Dr. Lucille, Dr. Lucille," she cried. "There's a young pregnant woman who went into labour twenty-four hours ago. It's her first child and I think the baby is lying crosswise in her stomach with its head on the left. I'm worried that we will need to operate to deliver her baby." Lucille examined the woman and found that she would indeed need a Caesarean delivery. "Could you show me where the operating theatre is?" she asked.

"Sorry, Doctor," Sister Anna replied. "We don't have one."

Lucille was in a panic. Her first thought was to pass the job to someone else. Then she remembered that there was no one else who could do it and that she was the only surgeon in the hospital. She asked the nurses to lay the patient on the table in a corner of the maternity unit and prepare her for the operation. Lucille then had another frightening thought: *I have never done a Caesarean operation!* She had observed them at medical school and had read about them in her textbooks but she had never actually performed the operation. For a split second, she was frozen with fear.

She knew that there was no alternative but to try. *"I know I have to do it,"* she told herself. She dashed over to the residence, dug out her medical textbooks, and quickly scanned the pages describing Caesarean deliveries. Then, still clutching a book, she returned to the patient. She scrubbed her hands, donned her rubber gloves, surgeon's cap, and mask while Piero gave the anesthetic. The textbook instructions swirled around in her head as she began the delicate operation.

"First, I am going to make an incision into the woman's abdomen so that I can move the baby's tiny head into position," Lucille explained as she precisely made the small incision. Then, very carefully, she reached in and slowly eased the baby out. The tiny body was all pink and greyish and covered in blood. Horrified, she thought, *My God, he's dead!* After a few seconds of anxious silence, the baby opened his mouth and gave a piercing squeal. It was the best sound she had ever heard.

The operation was a success. Lucille had delivered a healthy baby boy and the mother had come through it well. With a sigh of relief, she wiped the perspiration from her brow and collapsed in a chair.

Before she left that night, Lucille recorded details of the operation in the hospital's ledger, adding her initials, *L.T.* She had completed her first operation in Africa.

Lucille kept the young mother in the ward for several days to make sure there were no complications. When the woman was ready to leave, she wrapped her new baby in a shawl and slung him on her back. She then approached Lucille, cupped the doctor's hands in hers and said *"Apwoyo"* – "thank you" in her Acholi language. Lucille struggled to hold back her tears.

CO

Lucille's days were long and full. She spent most mornings checking the long line of outpatients who waited outside her small office. In the afternoon, she performed a non-stop succession of operations in her makeshift operating theatre, which was little more than a table and a single flickering light bulb. Drugs and antiseptics were scarce. There were so few instruments they often had to be re-sterilized during an operation. Conditions were, at best, basic.

"It seems as if all Africans are sick," Lucille wrote to her sister, Lise. "Most of them have malaria… It's difficult to care for the local people because you cannot question them. They do not know their age and they have no idea of time. They tell us that they have been sick for two weeks but it could have been two days or two years."

Lucille was also learning to adapt to a whole new life outside the hospital. She told her sister, "I don't eat as well as I did in Montreal, especially the meat. There is nothing but beef and chicken. On the other hand, we eat lots of vegetables (tomatoes, cucumbers, red peppers) and fruit (oranges, bananas, grapefruit, mangoes, papayas, which are a sort of melon which I don't like). At mealtime, we drink water with a touch of orange juice added. The one thing I really miss is milk. Oh yes, and maple syrup. And every night at about 10 p.m., we must turn out the lights since the electricity is cut off from 10 p.m. till 7 a.m."

On weekends, she and Piero went for walks in one of the national parks. In another letter to her sister, this time written by the glimmer of an oil lamp, she wrote, "On our last trip to the park, we stopped for a Coke and suddenly, just a hundred metres from where we were standing, there were about twenty hippos! They were splashing about in a pond and making so much noise with their huge mouths. We also watched in wonder as many giraffes and rhinos and several elephants loped past us."

While Lucille was adjusting to her new life, Piero spent much of his time seeking funds to build a new pediatric ward and an operating unit. He wrote dozens of letters in which he badgered friends and family, governments, and voluntary agencies to donate money and equipment. After almost six months his efforts paid off, and four military cargo planes arrived carrying ten tonnes of equipment into Uganda for the hospital.

�””⋄

Lucille became so caught up in her new life that her two-month stay stretched into four. Time passed quickly as she was enjoying her work and felt she was making a significant contribution. And she was growing accustomed and attached to Africa and its people.

She also enjoyed the time she spent with Piero. She loved driving off with him on weekend hunting trips, which in those days were a popular pastime, or going on safaris to one of the game parks. Everything was so new. So exciting.

However, Lucille still planned to finish her course in Marseilles, and she finally decided it was time to return to France. As the day of her departure approached, she realized more and more how much this new life had meant to her. It was also becoming clear to her that she had become very fond of Piero.

On the night before her departure, Piero took her aside and, holding her hand in his, he asked her to consider returning to Lacor. He had been looking for years for someone to share his dream, he said, someone to work with him in Africa and help him build a hospital that would be the finest in Uganda. "There's a lot of work to be done here, and we make a good team," he said. He paused, and added: "Besides, Lucille, I love you. I love you very much and I want you to marry me and stay here with me forever."

Lucille was stunned. Her first reaction was typical. "Are you mad?" she asked. "You cannot ask me to marry you just like that! It is much too quick. Anyway, remember that we had a deal. I came here for two months and it's already four. I'm leaving tomorrow."

"But Lucille," Piero begged. "If you do not know after four months, then you never will. Lucille, I love you."

Lucille needed more time to think. She had fully intended to finish her term in Marseilles, and then work for a period in child surgery in Paris so that she could obtain her diploma. She had even contemplated returning to work in Canada. Did she want to give this all up for a MAN? *No*, she thought. She would keep to her plan and return to Marseilles.

It was mid-September when Lucille packed her bags and prepared to leave. She walked through the wards for one last visit with some of her patients. She greeted a small child she had operated on the week before and offered a comforting word to his mother. She waved to a group of tiny children whom she had brought back to health and who would soon be returning home. Then, with a lump in her throat, she said goodbye to all the Sisters, hugging each one in turn. She climbed into the waiting car, and drove away.

Piero had decided to return home because his father was undergoing an operation in Italy. He suggested to Lucille that she meet him in Italy on her way back to France. She agreed to stop off in Rome so they could spend a few days together. Piero met her at the Rome airport with a bouquet of red roses. They spent three days visiting the famous sights of Rome before travelling together to Besana to visit Piero's family.

The family welcomed Lucille like one of their own. Piero was now thirty-five and his parents had almost despaired of his ever marrying. They saw in Lucille the perfect wife for their son. For her part, Lucille felt much more comfortable with them than she had on her earlier visit. But she was still not ready to commit herself.

At the station platform in Milan, Piero took Lucille's hands in his and said: "Lucille, I want to offer you my thanks for all your help and support these past few months." Then he paused, gathered his courage and asked her again, "Will you marry me?"

As she stepped aboard the train, she gave him a cryptic reply. "I promise you that one day we will see each other again in Gulu." They kissed goodbye and she left for Marseilles.

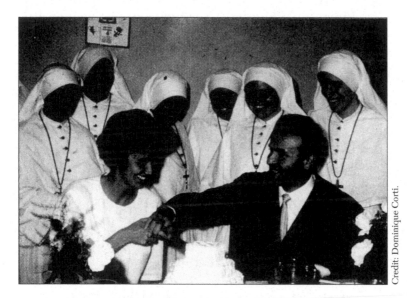

Credit: Dominique Corti.

Surrounded by the Comboni nuns, Lucille and Piero cut
their wedding cake following their marriage in December 1961.

4

Return to Uganda

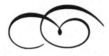

We are the only doctors here and we work without much rest from morning till evening. The needs are so great. We do just about everything, from pediatrics to malaria and wounds inflicted by elephants and lions.
— Lucille Teasdale, January 1962

Lucille was glad to be back with her friends at the hospital. Yet as she slotted back into her earlier routine, she found it hard to concentrate on her work. Every minute of the day, she found herself thinking about Piero and about the time they had spent together in Uganda. She missed him terribly and finally admitted to herself that she had fallen in love with him and wanted to share the rest of her life with him.

Piero was still in Italy but about to leave for Uganda. Lucille telephoned him the night before his departure. "I am calling to give you my answer," she explained.

There was a brief pause while Lucille tried to remain calm. "The answer is yes," she said. "Yes" she would marry him and "yes," she would return to live with him in Africa. Piero was ecstatic.

Lucille had never been happier. She was deeply in love and thought about Piero constantly. She wrote to him almost daily in carefully penned letters written on flimsy aerograms.

"How can I carry on without you?" she wrote. "... I have decided I do not want to do anything without you. I love you, Piero. I need you." And later, she said: "Do you remember the day I left you at the station and you thanked me? Well, it is I who must thank you for having saved me from myself, from a life of solitude. You have given me so much happiness. You are such a good person, much better than I. I hope that, with time, I will become worthy of you."

In order to feel closer to Piero, Lucille began to go to Mass again. "I did it, not yet by conviction, but because it brought me closer to you. It was also very nice to sit and think of you without any distractions." In a later letter, in a surprising revelation of her feelings of inadequacy, she confided: "Piero, I am not the strong, independent and cold woman that I have given the impression of all these years. I am a little girl who has forgotten to grow up, a little girl who has finally found someone who can take her hand and walk with her through life. If you only knew how helpless I am without you."

The flurry of letters continued. Piero was now back in Uganda, and when he had finished his long day's work in the hospital, he would sit down and share his thoughts with Lucille. On 5 October, he wrote: "All I want is to love you Lucille. To have you by my side during my life's journey, to have you beside me in the hospital, in my home, in my car, in my bed, to live with you for the rest of my life."

During this period, Lucille became consumed with the idea of motherhood. "No one wants a child more than I, and how I long for you to be the father of my children," she wrote to Piero. "But I have always had a great fear that a child of mine might have the same awful feelings towards me that I had towards my own mother... Often I wonder if it is better to abandon the idea of motherhood for fear of having children who would hate me..."

As the weeks progressed, Lucille decided to withdraw from her course in Marseilles. She also went to Paris to cancel her internship. During the meeting, her professor used the occasion to challenge her decision. Why are you giving up the position? Why are you leaving France? What country are you going to? What type of medicine will you be doing there? She became so flustered by all the questions that she burst into tears. The same night, she wrote to Piero: "For many years, I did not know how to cry," she admitted. "I tried to convince myself that it was not a good thing to cry, but now I believe that deep down, I missed out on something. I believe that you can live more intensely when you are able to be moved, even by small things. It is through you, Piero, that I have rediscovered the soul of my childhood."

⚭

Piero telephoned his family to tell them about his engagement, and they called Lucille at once to ask her to visit them in Besana. They would not be able to attend the wedding, they told her, as it would be taking place in Uganda, so they insisted on having a party to celebrate the event. Piero could not leave Uganda to join the party, but a telegram awaited Lucille's arrival in Besana. "Welcome to our home STOP Mama, papa, brothers and sisters all welcome you STOP Impossible to live without you STOP Come Piero."

Lucille was still nervous visiting the family, especially without Piero. "I still feel like a misfit when I am with your family," she told him. "I have tried to escape from my working-class background but I have not yet managed to feel comfortable in the more refined surroundings that you have grown up in. In some ways, I still feel like the little factory worker from our east end neighbourhood. I guess that is why I like the French singer, Edith Piaf, so much. To hear this little woman pour out her grief always brings tears to my eyes."

Nonetheless, Lucille soon began to feel more comfortable with Piero's family. His sister Angela became a special friend and took her shopping to buy their wedding rings. "I chose ones in yellow gold," she told Piero. "I had forgotten to ask your advice so I hope you will like them."

Their shopping spree did not stop there. "Angela wanted me to buy some nightgowns. I cannot bring myself to tell her that I do not want any, that I want to sleep with you just as God made me! And she could not imagine how we could possibly live without beautiful embroidered sheets. When I have the good fortune to have a Piero, I don't need anything else!"

Angela also took Lucille on a sightseeing trip to Lago Maggiore. "Oh Piero, how I love Italy and the Italians! Remember how I worried how I would manage in long discussions in Italian? Now I love to try and speak the language. It is almost like music for me. Every day, I am beginning to feel more and more Italian."

The engagement party was held in Besana, in October 1961, and the whole family – Piero's brothers and sisters and all their children – assembled at the Corti home, which was overflowing with red roses sent by Piero. He had asked his mother to buy an engagement ring for Lucille so, during the party, she called for silence, took Lucille's hand in hers and solemnly slipped the ring on her finger. Everyone burst into applause. Then she read another telegram that arrived from Piero. It read "On our engagement day Lucille in Besana and me in Gulu!"

Lucille felt overwhelmed by the family's affection for her. She found Piero's mother to be an especially caring person and could not help but compare her to her own mother. "Happily I did not have a mother like yours," she wrote to Piero after the party "because I would never have been able to marry you. I would never have wanted to live far away from her. Piero, if we ever have children, you must help me to become a mother like yours.

"Thank you, Piero, for giving me, as well as your love, a real family, one which I only imagined but never believed existed."

Lucille left the next day for Montreal. She was anxious to share her news with her own family, especially her father. When she told them about her engagement to Piero, they all embraced her warmly. She then decided to splurge for such a big occasion, so she visited the best shop in town and spent one hundred dollars on a wedding dress. It was a very simple model, white with a black corsage. When she described the new dress to Piero's sister, Angela was aghast. "Your wedding dress must be all white," she said. "But don't worry. I will have an all-white one made for you in Milan."

Lucille's stay in Montreal was not easy. "Unfortunately, I find my mother increasingly more difficult," she wrote to Piero. "I like being with Papa but I do not like being with my mother. My happiest times here have been in the morning when I do errands with my father..." As before, Lucille did not feel she could confide in her father, but she believed he understood that these hours alone with him were precious to her, for she would be sacrificing future time with him when she joined Piero in Africa.

By late-November, Lucille had finished all the preparations for her departure and was ready to leave Canada. She flew first to Milan, where Piero's family gave her more gifts – sheets, pillowcases, napkins – which they called "Piero's trousseau." Angela presented her with a beautiful wedding dress, very simple and all white. She also gave her a white lace veil made in a factory near their family home.

Lucille was very touched by the family's kindness and said she did not know how to thank them. "But Lucille," said Piero's mother. "It is we who must thank you." The next day, the whole family gathered at the airport to see her off. She embraced each one in turn and boarded the plane for Africa.

⌖

Lucille arrived back in Africa on 4 December 1961 in a state of great excitement. She was returning for good to live among the people she had come to respect, to the work she had found so satisfying and rewarding. Above all, she was returning to marry the man she loved, to make a home with him.

Piero met her at the airport in his convertible Volkswagen Beetle. The meeting was a joyful one. After two months' separation, they hugged and kissed each other as never before. At long last, they were together again.

Lucille had said that she wanted to marry as soon as possible after her arrival, and Piero had taken her at her word. He had made the wedding arrangements for the following morning, which meant that they had to reach Gulu by nightfall to finish all the preparations.

There was no time to lose. Piero piled Lucille's luggage into the car, and they set out on the long journey north. "It was a terrible day with torrential rains," Lucille recalled. "The main road was completely flooded, so we had to take a much longer route, navigating around deep pools of water and mud. We had three flat tires on the way, so we didn't reach the hospital until after midnight."

They barely slept that night and woke at dawn to prepare for the wedding that morning. The ceremony was set for 8 a.m., and according to Lucille's wishes it would take place in the chapel on the grounds of the hospital. The Comboni Sisters had decorated the chapel with red hibiscus flowers and white orange blossoms. They had even searched the region for a rose bush so that the bride could carry a bouquet of red roses.

The chapel was packed with well-wishers. The Sisters sat in the front pews, and the Ugandan nurses filled the benches behind them. There was a long wait before Piero arrived at the chapel. Then, a few minutes later, Lucille entered, dressed in her white wedding dress with the Italian lace veil draped over her head and shoulders.

The ceremony was a simple one led by the Bishop of Gulu. The couple solemnly exchanged their marriage vows, and then Piero lifted Lucille's wedding veil and kissed her. When they left the chapel, the guests showered the couple with handfuls of rice, while the Sisters burst into song and clapped their hands. Everyone moved on to the dining room for a wedding breakfast of bacon and eggs.

The nuns had made a three-tiered wedding cake and passed around pieces to each guest. They opened a bottle of red Cinzano, an Italian vermouth, and everyone drank a toast to the newlyweds, to the hospital, and to Uganda. They also drank a toast to Italy, for Lucille, through her marriage to Piero, had now become a citizen of his country.

After the ceremony, Lucille and Piero prepared to leave for a ten-day honeymoon in neighbouring Kenya. But first, Lucille had one obligation to fulfil: still wearing her wedding dress, she donned her white medical coat and made the rounds of the whole hospital ward. She had been absent for three months and wanted to check on each of the patients before leaving.

The couple set off by car on the long journey to Nairobi, where they boarded a plane for Zanzibar, an island in the Indian Ocean off the coast of what is today called Tanzania.

Lucille and Piero found the island, "very romantic" and they spent many long hours swimming in the sea or walking hand in hand along the white sandy beaches that bordered the Indian Ocean. They were deliriously happy to be together and savoured these moments of calm.

∽

When they returned from their honeymoon, the couple moved into a small house in the compound. In no time, they were both back on the job working side-by side all day and often well into the night. While Piero handled most of the administrative matters as well as any anesthetic duties, Lucille started her day by examining up to three hundred outpatients in a morning. Malaria was the most common disease, but many suffered from pneumonia or other respiratory ailments, malnourishment or dysentery. Lucille also interviewed at least twenty new admissions each day and helped vaccinate hundreds of young children to protect them from tropical diseases.

As she worked, Lucille would talk at top speed, switching effortlessly from English to French, or from Italian to her newly learned Acholi, the local language. She worked with the same intensity. "In the time it takes most people to examine one patient, Lucille can see five," said her proud husband.

Lucille spent the afternoons doing surgery, usually with Piero at her side to help with the anesthetics. Operations varied from repairing a ruptured appendix or removing a tumour to delivering a baby, often in the middle of the night.

Lucille turned out to be a masterful surgeon. She worked quickly and precisely and she directed her team of nurses like an orchestra conductor. During an operation, she insisted on absolute silence from the nurses. They must never disturb her, must never cross their arms. All the staff had to maintain her high standards of cleanliness and follow her orders meticulously. These were things she had learned during her work in Canada and in France, and she was determined to pass them on so that her staff would be trained to be thorough and efficient.

The conditions she worked under were unlike anything she had seen before. There was still no operating room, so they installed a few lamps and continued to use a makeshift operating table built from a homemade bed. Electricity was sporadic and a clean water supply was not always available. There was only the most rudimentary equipment and always a shortage of drugs. Even though the number of children who required surgery was increasing, there was still no pediatric ward. Children who required surgery were lumped in with all the other patients.

Her tasks were daunting under such conditions, but Lucille was up to the challenge. "We are the only doctors here and we work without much rest from morning till evening," she wrote to her sister. "The needs are so great. We do just about everything, from pediatrics to malaria and wounds inflicted by elephants and lions. Piero is constantly begging for money and supplies. We lack everything, but that will never stand in our way…"

Both Lucille and Piero seemed oblivious to the many obstacles they faced.

They were happy in their work, they were happy to be doing it together, and they found much satisfaction in taking the first small steps toward turning the hospital into a first-class facility.

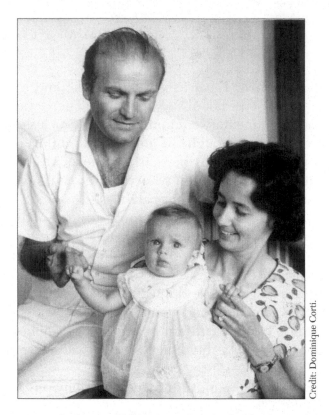

The happy family soon after the birth of
Dominique. "We have been blessed with a baby
girl," Lucille wrote to her sisters.

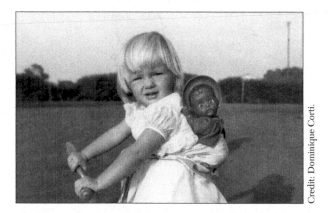

Dominique carries her baby doll
in the African manner.

5

Birth of a Country – and a Baby Daughter

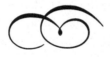

*We have been blessed with a baby girl.
Dominique was born on Saturday night. I rested
on Sunday and worked again on Monday.*
Lucille Teasdale, 17 November 1962

On 9 October 1962, Uganda finally gained its independence from Britain.

The day was one of great celebration. In towns and villages throughout the country, people danced and sang. In the capital, members of the British royal family presided over a glittering ceremony. They watched from their Royal Box as two military officers stepped up to a flagpole and slowly lowered the Union Jack.

Before a cheering crowd, the officers then raised the new flag of Uganda – a crested crane wearing a crown against a background of stripes of black (for Africa), yellow (for the sun), and red (for solidarity). As it flapped in the breeze, a choir of schoolchildren sang Uganda's new national anthem.

The people of Uganda retained the British Governor General, but they appointed a Ugandan president, Sir Edward Mutesa, a member of the Baganda tribe, the principal tribe in the south of the country. Real power, however, passed into the hands of the newly appointed Prime Minister, Milton Obote, who came from the north of the country.

This was a utopian period for Uganda. The economy was booming, thanks to an abundance of coffee and cotton, sugar and tea, and to the proceeds of its large copper mines. The capital, Kampala, was a thriving and prosperous city. Its shops were filled with imported goods and markets overflowed with a wide variety of locally grown fruits and vegetables.

Above all, Uganda was a tourist paradise. Visitors flocked to the land from countries around the world. They came to enjoy the agreeable climate and breathtaking scenery and to visit the game parks to watch herds of wild animals – antelopes and zebras, lions and giraffes – that roamed the plains. There was optimism for the future. And there was peace.

∞

For Lucille and Piero, the work continued, and they managed to do wonders with limited outside assistance.

Gradually, they were able to attract several Italian doctors who chose to do their internship at St. Mary's, now renamed St. Mary's-Lacor or just Lacor Hospital. More importantly, they began to recruit Ugandan medical interns from Makerere University in Kampala, who came to them for their surgical training.

Their daily routine seldom changed. Lucille was up by 7 a.m. every morning. She had breakfast with Piero, then walked across the lawn to the hospital and began her rounds.

Each day, she started in a different ward. She assembled all the doctors to discuss the cases they were dealing with. Together, they reviewed the progress of each patient to decide whether the treatment had worked, whether it should be changed, or whether the patient could be discharged.

As she walked through the ward, Lucille looked every inch the doctor: she wore a long white medical coat, her stethoscope dangled from her neck, and glasses perched on her nose. She would greet each patient in Acholi, then fire off questions, sometimes with the help of an interpreter. How does this boy feel? Has he been vomiting for long? How are we treating this man? What are we doing for this woman's fever?

At about 11 a.m., Lucille would take a short break, then return to deal with the long line of outpatients. A nurse who spoke their own language first interviewed them and noted the details on a chart. Lucille would then examine them and decide whether they should be admitted to the hospital or whether they could receive treatment as an outpatient. It was a real assembly-line operation.

"Bring in Mr. Ayama," she would shout. A young man would shuffle in complaining of a headache, fever, and shivering. She would take his temperature, check his blood pressure, and look over his chart. "Malaria," Lucille would say to the attending nurse. "Give him chloroquine. Next please." This woman appears to have had a duodenal ulcer and has been in pain for ten years. "Ten years?" Lucille would ask, shaking her head in frustration. "Admit her at once and check her more thoroughly," she would say, moving on to the next patient without skipping a beat. During a typical morning, Lucille would see as many as two hundred patients.

Once a patient was admitted, they would be asked if they had brought along a *lagwok*, usually a wife or mother, who would live in the "parent's quarters" and help care for the patient and do their cooking. The *lagwoks* would sleep in the courtyard, often with their sisters or aunts and children in tow.

By 2 p.m., Lucille would walk home for lunch and a short rest before returning to the hospital for the long afternoon in the operating room. Before the first operation, she would spend at least ten minutes scrubbing her arms and hands with soap and a brush, then put on a green long-sleeved gown, a surgeon's cap and mask, and plastic gloves. For simple operations, she would do the anesthetic herself, usually an "epidural." For more complicated operations, she would call on Piero to give the anesthetic and he would stay to monitor the patient during the operation.

Occasionally, Lucille would be stymied by a case or uncertain about her ability to carry out a particularly difficult operation. "I just can't do this," she would admit to Piero. "It is just too complicated." They would discuss the case together, Piero would give some suggestions, and then she would return to work, with Piero at her elbow to offer encouragement.

Lucille seldom finished operating before 8 p.m. While the nuns prepared her some fresh juice – orange, lemon, and tamarind were favourites – she would sit at a desk and jot down details of all the operations she had performed that day. She rarely reached home before 9 p.m.

A local cook who had been trained by the nuns prepared dinner and Lucille was happy to hand over the kitchen to him. She never enjoyed housekeeping, much less cooking, and she would only rarely take down her frayed French Canadian cookbook on the cook's day off. "My specialties are chocolate pudding and crème caramel. That's about it," she laughed. She would read for an hour and was more than ready for bed by 11.30 p.m.

∞

Their first year was a period of great satisfaction for Lucille and Piero. They were able to establish a routine that suited them both, and Lucille, especially, found her job rewarding. As word about the new doctor at Lacor Hospital spread around the region, patients began to arrive in droves. Many came from as far as one hundred kilometres away, and most travelled on foot. One patient, who had broken both his legs, was pushed into the hospital in a wheelbarrow. The journey from his home had taken them three days.

Each day brought new challenges. One of the most difficult Lucille had to face was how to deal with some of the tribal customs practised in her new land. Soon after her arrival, she noticed that many small babies were brought in with a strange infection in their gums, a condition their mothers called *ebino*, which resulted from an ancient custom practised in many of the villages in the north.

When a baby became ill and feverish and there was swelling around the canine teeth – the sharp, pointed teeth near the front of the mouth – the mother would immediately take the child to an *ajwaka*, a village healer. The *ajwaka* would make incisions in the baby's gums with the tip of an arrow or an old bicycle spoke and extract the canine teeth. Most children managed to recover but many others would succumb to serious infection or tetanus. Occasionally, the child would bleed to death.

One day, when Lucille was examining a patient, there was a knock on the door. In stepped a young woman carrying her small baby on her back. The child's face was strangely disfigured: her lower gums were swollen and she hardly had the strength to open her eyes. The tiny body was shivering and she was breathing heavily through her mouth. Clearly, the child was close to death.

"What happened to her?" Lucille asked the mother. The woman looked down and mumbled in a barely audible whisper. "*Ebino*."

Lucille was furious. She was angry with the mother. "Why did you wait so long before bringing your child to the hospital?" she asked. She was also angry with the Acholi people for allowing themselves to be victims of a dangerous tradition that often led to the pointless death of many of their babies.

Lucille examined the baby carefully before making her diagnosis. "She has acute infectious osteomyelitis, a serious inflammation of the bone marrow," Lucille explained to the mother. Cupping the tiny face in her hands, she continued. "Part of the baby's lower jawbone is infected," she said. "It is clear that the tissue is already dead and will probably lead to gangrene."

Not surprisingly, the child had been unable to swallow for several days. Lucille inserted a tube through her nose in order to feed her and gave her a dose of antibiotics. In spite of all her efforts, the baby died.

During her stay in Uganda, Lucille had learned to understand and to respect many of the local customs. However, when the traditional ways were clearly life-threatening, as was the Acholi people's treatment of *ebino*, she felt it was important to point out the dangers of some of these practices. "You are killing your babies by doing this," she told the mothers. "This custom can so easily lead to a serious infection, especially if you do not see a doctor at once." Then she added, "A baby died just last week because her mother left it so long to bring her to the hospital." She was hoping that, by citing this example, she might teach them an important lesson.

∞

Lucille and Piero spent most of their weekends in the countryside. Piero had always been passionate about hunting, and Lucille would often join him on hunting expeditions or a trip to a game reserve in one of the nearby national parks. These outings were their only break, and they delighted in setting out to explore the region.

In the first spring of their busy new life together, Lucille was thrilled to discover she was pregnant. She had always hoped to have children, but she had already suffered a miscarriage. Now that she was pregnant again, friends tried to encourage her to reduce her heavy workload. Lucille would have none of it. "Why should I slow down?" she asked them. "Pregnancy is not an illness." She insisted on continuing her hectic schedule, though she did take more frequent breaks.

Luckily, her pregnancy went well. One Saturday in November, while she was at work, her contractions began. She still refused to leave the hospital until she had finished her rounds. By the time Piero finally called her gynecologist to help with the delivery, it was too late. Lucille had already gone into labour and, after two and a half hours, with the help of both Piero and a midwife, she gave birth to a baby daughter.

They named their new baby Dominique. When their Acholi friends heard the news, they gave the baby another name: *Atim*, meaning "born in a foreign land." From then on, Lucille became known as *Min Atim* or mother of *Atim*.

Lucille and Piero were overjoyed with their baby. Lucille wrote at once to share the news with her sisters in Montreal. "We have been blessed with a baby girl. Dominique was born on Saturday night," she told them. "I rested on Sunday and started work again on Monday!" It seemed quite natural for her to return to work so soon. She had often seen the Acholi women working in the fields barely twenty-four hours after giving birth. Lucille saw no reason why she should be any different.

Little Dominique's life was a happy one. She was looked after by her Acholi *lapidi* (nanny), Liberata, who shared Dominique's room until she was four and always spoke to her in Acholi. Liberata would carry the baby on her back wrapped in a shawl, just as African mothers did.

Dominique grew to become a blonde, blue-eyed child who scampered freely around the hospital compound. She was surrounded by different languages and absorbed them all. She learned French from her parents, Italian from both her father and the nuns, and English at school. But Acholi was her first language. "All the children she plays with are Ugandan, and they all speak Acholi together," laughed Lucille. "Very often, she quite unconsciously speaks Acholi with us!"

Dominique felt right at home in her African surroundings. She had many African friends, and she also loved animals. Her favourite animal friend was a gazelle that she fed milk to with a baby's bottle. One day, she and her parents came home to find the gazelle lying in its pen, dead. Dominique was devastated and cried uncontrollably. "How long has the animal been dead?" Lucille asked Liberata.

"For at least two hours," she replied.

"But why did you not hide the body and tell Dominique the animal had run away? Why did you leave the carcass here?"

"Because, doctor," Liberata explained, "death is a part of life, and children, even young ones, must learn to understand that." Lucille had to admit that although she was often quick to denounce Acholi customs, some of them did show much wisdom.

Even before Dominique began school, she would often stay with Lucille in the hospital. At first, she would sit in a corner of the room with a colouring book, but later, she liked to follow her mother on her rounds.

∞

Dominique started attending the local school when she was six. In the first grades, the lessons were all given in Acholi, but as they progressed, the children began to learn English. Dominique loved school. She was the only white child among the hundreds of black children, but her teachers assured Lucille and Piero that she felt perfectly at home.

Dominique also loved Sunday – the special day of the week when she joined her parents on a journey to one of the national parks. Piero and one or two of his friends would spend the day hunting for antelopes or warthogs while Lucille and Dominique would go for long walks or have a swim. They would return home late the same evening.

As the number of patients at the hospital increased each month, Lucille and Piero managed to receive help from Italian doctors and interns. But they quickly realized that if their hospital was to fully succeed, their top priority must be to educate Ugandan doctors and nurses.

They began by setting up a training program for nurses. The Canadian government provided a grant of

$240,000, and in 1973, Lucille and Piero opened the Lacor Nursing Training School, a handsome new school and residence for student nurses. This was the first nursing school outside Kampala, and it provided space for seventy-two students to follow a three-year course.

The first graduation ceremony was held on the outside lawn. That day twenty-five young nurses filed onto the grounds, each one proudly wearing her bright blue uniform and starched white cap. As the graduates stepped forward to accept their diplomas, Lucille and Piero watched from the front row, beaming like proud parents. They devised similar courses for health educators, midwives, laboratory technicians, and radiographers.

Another of Lucille and Piero's priorities was to make health care available to those living in far-distant villages, so they built a network of three small clinics in remote corners of the region. Community health teams, including midwives and health educators who had been trained at Lacor, would visit these centres each week to offer health education, especially to mothers, and run wide-scale vaccination programs for children. Through these satellite clinics, thousands of children were able to feel the presence of the hospital.

Already, Lucille and Piero had begun to realize many of their dreams.

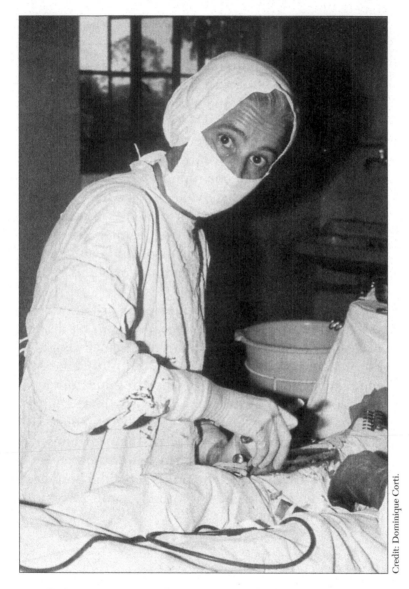

Lucille becomes a war surgeon. During these turbulent years, she performs more than 1000 operations to treat gunshot wounds.

6

A Wily Dictator Seizes Power

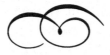

Your father and I have two children. One is weak and the other is strong. The hospital is our weak child. We cannot abandon it now.
– Lucille Teasdale, September 1972

Lucille and Piero continued to do everything possible to expand and improve the hospital. They raised funds to erect new buildings and solicited donations of medical equipment, largely from the Italian government. They enjoyed the challenge of looking for ways to build a bigger and better hospital. "For somebody in our profession, this is the most rewarding place you could ever hope to be," Lucille wrote to her sisters. "We can do anything we like."

But as they were searching for ways and means to improve the hospital, there were ominous developments elsewhere in the country. At the time of independence, Uganda already faced divisions among its many tribes. The country was primarily polarized between northerners and southerners. The new prime minister, Milton Obote, who came from the north of the country, tried his best to unite the different factions, but the divisions were deep-seated and proved impossible to resolve. When Obote decided to oust the president, who was from the southern Baganda tribe, this large and powerful tribe turned against him. He tried to crush them, but the move lit the fuse that would lead to his own destruction.

The prime minister needed the support of the army, so he turned to one of his senior military officers for help. The officer was Lieutenant Colonel Idi Amin, whom he soon promoted to Commander of the army. Amin was a Moslem with a fierce loyalty to his small Kakwa tribe from the northwest. There was widespread hope that he could stabilize the army, but under his direction, the armed forces too became dangerously divided.

In late January, 1971, Prime Minister Obote left Uganda to attend a conference of Commonwealth prime ministers and presidents in Singapore. He expected to be home within a week.

On January 25, Amin and his fellow conspirators seized the occasion to overthrow the government. In one sweeping move, Amin declared himself Uganda's new president.

Idi Amin was forty-six. He was a mountain of a man, a chunky six feet tall and a former heavyweight boxing champion with an earthy, barrack-style sense of humour. From the start, he ruled like the military officer he was. He had assumed supreme power and called himself Idi Amin Dada, adding the title "President for Life."

In his first speech to the nation, Amin promised to transfer power to a civilian government as soon as elections could be organized. Ugandans were relieved. Most thought that he would make a good president. They prayed that he would unite Uganda and bring peace and prosperity to the land.

Their hopes were soon to be shattered. Barely weeks after Amin took control of the government, it became apparent that he was in fact a power-hungry tyrant. He suspended all political activities and ordered the army to shoot anyone suspected of opposing his regime.

Suddenly, people began to disappear. Amin's soldiers seized any rivals or potential rivals to the president and dragged them away, never to be seen again. Amin turned first upon the professional classes and ordered the elimination of cabinet ministers, university professors – anyone who could be seen as a threat to him. The army chief of staff "disappeared." The vice-rector of Makerere University "disappeared." Soldiers acting on Amin's orders arrested the country's chief justice and murdered him in broad daylight. Then they targeted Christians and Jews. The Protestant archbishop was another victim.

As the carnage spread, entire villages populated by tribes who had supported Milton Obote were simply wiped out. "At the time, we did not quite understand what was happening," Lucille recalled later. "But it wasn't long before the true nature of the military government began to show."

In fact, the insidious work of the military government had only just begun. In a move that horrified both Ugandans and the international community, Amin announced, on 4 August 1972, that he was expelling the 70,000 Asians, mostly of Indian origin, who lived in Uganda. They included businessmen, lawyers, engineers, administrators, and doctors – people who were the backbone of the country's commercial sector. They were given ninety days to leave and could carry little more than the clothes they wore. Amin promised to give their jobs and their property to African businessmen. Instead, he handed these over to his own military henchmen.

The military and the heavily armed police force continued their campaign of terror. Prisons were overflowing. Thousands of innocent Ugandans were taken without warning and killed at whim. By 1979, an estimated 300,000 people – one Ugandan in every forty – had died.

With each passing year, the country slid deeper into chaos. Amin suspected that the Acholis in the north were loyal to Obote, so they became targets of his terror squads. Since Lacor Hospital lay in Acholi territory, it was often caught in the crossfire.

Lucille and Piero had little choice but to carry on despite the upheavals. There was fighting all around them, and a never-ending influx of wounded soldiers found their way to the hospital. Almost before she knew what was happening, Dr. Lucille had become a war surgeon.

∞

The vast majority of the patients who were arriving at the hospital had received gunshot wounds. The most lethal were the "soft bullets" that buried themselves in the flesh and exploded within the body, leaving a mass of bone fragments as sharp as razor blades. About 90 per cent of Lucille's work required her to deal with the damage inflicted by these insidious soft bullets.

Lucille found that the best way to clean such wounds was to reach inside and pluck out the shards of bone with her fingers. As she probed inside a damaged limb to retrieve bone fragments, she would often cut her fingers on the sharp edges of bone that would puncture the two pairs of rubber gloves she had taken to wearing. Whenever she cut herself, she would remove her gloves immediately, disinfect her hands, put on a new double pair and carry on with the operation. Often, she would change her gloves four or five times during a single operation. About her own health, she was fearless. She had a job to do and nothing was going to stop her caring for those in need, whatever the risk to her.

The days were long and hard. By nighttime, Lucille cherished her only chance to relax. She would return to her house with Piero, sip a glass of home-made wine, and listen to records of their favourite singers, such as Frank Sinatra, on an old RCA wind-up record player. Their home was their only refuge in a world gone mad.

∞

As the fighting continued to escalate around them, Lucille rarely stopped to think about her own safety. But she did become increasingly concerned about the safety of nine-year-old Dominique. There was no question that they would keep the hospital open and continue to serve the local population, who needed them more than ever. But what about Dominique? Was it wise to keep her here when they were living on such a powder keg?

Lucille had always vowed that she would never be separated from her daughter. But despite her strong feelings about keeping the family together, she could no longer ignore the growing danger. Piero also felt that Dominique needed a more challenging education than the one she could receive in the small local school. With huge misgivings, they made the painful decision to send Dominique to Italy, where she would live with Piero's sister and attend a nearby school run by the Ursuline Sisters.

The decision was particularly hard for Lucille. She was consumed with feelings of guilt and feared that Dominique might feel that her mother did not love her, just as Lucille herself had felt unloved by her own mother. At first, Dominique appeared to accept the decision. Later, she asked her parents: "Why can't you come with me to Italy?"

Lucille tried to explain: "Your father and I have two children. One is weak and the other is strong. The hospital is our weak child. We cannot abandon it now."

A month later, when the day of departure arrived, Lucille and Piero drove Dominique to the airport. The couple chatted nervously, trying to console their daughter while they hid their own anxiety. At the airport, Lucille fought hard to hold back tears as she gave her daughter a final hug. Then, with a wave, she watched the tiny figure climb aboard the plane.

∞

They returned to the hospital and Lucille immersed herself in her work with twice her previous zeal. She had told her daughter that the hospital needed her, and she was determined to meet that need. As the number of surgery cases mounted, she started operating on two patients at a time. She would finish one, hand the patient over to an intern, change her gloves, and start on the next. She worked faster than ever before, not wanting to leave anyone unattended. Her personal record was completing a Caesarean operation in twenty-three minutes rather than the normal hour or more!

She also worked with new-found confidence and no longer felt she needed Piero's help when she encountered a particularly complicated case. Instead, she simply told herself that she could do what was required and would jump right in.

In the operating room, Lucille showed the skill of a seasoned surgeon. She worked quickly and with deep concentration and would often barely notice the time. Occasionally, Piero would see that her rubber gloves were torn or punctured so that her hands were in contact with a patient's blood. "Lucille," he would remind her in his own meticulous way, "you must always remember to change your gloves between operations."

Lucille would reply with the same answer: she knew that she risked getting a disease such as hepatitis B or an infection called septicemia, but both these could be easily cured with antibiotics. "Surgeons are always taking risks," she pointed out. "That is part of our profession."

Though her work was all-consuming, Lucille missed Dominique very much. She thought of her daughter morning and night and between operations. Each day, she hoped for a letter from her daughter, but she heard nothing until three months after Dominique had left.

My dear Mama and Papa,

This is the first letter that I am writing to you. I am still young and I do not know how to tell you many things. I promise that I will not be naughty and that I will always be kind and obedient. I wish you a very happy Christmas.

Your daughter,
Dominique

Lucille burst into tears. She had dreamed of spending Christmas with her daughter, but she knew it was impossible for them to leave the hospital and travel to Italy. She also knew it was unsafe for Dominique to come to visit them. She had never imagined that she would have to spend Christmas separated from her child.

Dominique stayed on at the school in Italy, even though she was very homesick. In one letter, she asked her parents if she could come back to live with them "otherwise I will die!" And in another: "When I get up in the morning, I ask myself why isn't my mother here to wake me up with a kiss? Why do I have to wake up by a stupid alarm clock? I do not want to stay here any longer."

Lucille was devastated to learn that Dominique was so unhappy. They had sent her away with the best intentions, but clearly, it had not worked as they had hoped. Something had to be done.

She and Piero discussed alternatives. "If Dominique does not want to stay there without us, then we must go and stay there with her," Lucille said firmly. "We will find some other doctors to replace us at the hospital."

Piero was not so sure. Certainly Dominique was very precious to them but so was the hospital. "I think we should let Dominique decide," he said.

They telephoned Dominique. "If you would like us to come to Italy to be with you, we are ready to do so," said Lucille.

"Oh, no," Dominique replied. That is out of the question. You do not need to come to Italy. I will come to Africa."

They explained that the situation in Uganda was still too dangerous. "Then I could go to a boarding school in Kenya." This sounded like a good idea to Lucille. One of Piero's sisters lived in Nairobi, so Dominique could spend weekends with her aunt and visit her parents in Uganda at the end of each term. It was settled, and Dominique flew to Kenya in time to start school the following term.

∽

Dominique loved her new school. She studied hard, got good marks, and was thrilled to have the chance to take riding lessons, a passion she was to pursue for many years. Almost at once, her letters took on a different tone.

Dear Mama and Papa,

I have now found a moment to write to you. I have just finished my riding lesson and I still have the taste of wheat and barley in my mouth... Today, we took all the horses out, with me in the lead... I have also learned to jump a barrier...

Dominique returned to Gulu every three months. She enjoyed coming back to the home she had loved as a child, to her own room still filled with her childhood books and mementoes. She especially looked forward to helping Lucille in the hospital, giving vaccinations in the children's dispensary, or sterilizing instruments in the operating room. Lucille and Piero were happy that their daughter was showing an interest in the hospital. It was their hope that some day she would decide to study medicine and perhaps come to work with them at Lacor. They even dared to think that as they grew older, she might some day want to take over their responsibilities.

That was all a distant dream. For the moment, as the country continued to sink into chaos, Lucille and Piero had their hands full just keeping the hospital functioning.

In a quiet moment at the end of a long working day in April 1974, Lucille sat down and wrote to Lise. "It was thirteen years ago today that I arrived in Uganda. Who would have thought that I would have stayed this long! When we arrived, there was a tiny hospital of 40 beds and a small dispensary. Now there are 205 beds, two dispensaries, a laboratory (one of the best in Uganda) and a radiology department, also one of the best in Uganda. I think we can well be proud of what we have done.

"If sometimes we think of leaving here," she continued, "we have to stop and think about who could replace us and keep the hospital running at the same level of efficiency." Lucille knew that this was the stark reality. So far, there was no one who could fill their shoes. But for the moment, Lucille and Piero had more immediate concerns.

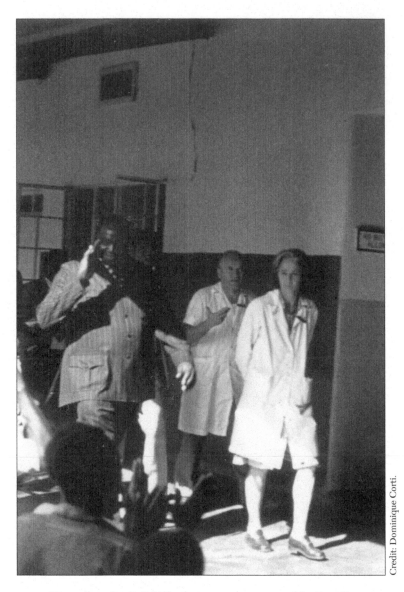

"President for Life" Idi Amin is accompanied by Lucille
and Piero during a visit to Lacor Hospital.

7

The Carnage Continues

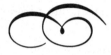

> *How can we go on living and working under*
> *these conditions? I know for the moment that we*
> *have no choice. We are the only doctors in the*
> *whole region so we must stay.*
> — Lucille Teasdale, 15 May 1979

The ugly shadow of Idi Amin blanketed the whole country in fear. The mere mention of his name caused people to tremble as rumours of his heavy-handed brutality spread far and wide. Soldiers arriving at Lacor Hospital brought stories of army barracks that doubled as torture chambers where Amin incarcerated his victims and bludgeoned them to death with sledge-hammers.

Amin rarely travelled around the country, so a late-night phone call to Piero one evening in 1976 came as a shock. Piero had just gone to bed and was only half awake as the caller explained that he was from the office of the president and that Idi Amin himself would be travelling to the northern region and wished to visit Lacor Hospital.

Piero was stunned. Imagine the country's president wanting to visit the hospital! He caught his breath and managed to reply. "Well, of course," he answered, still fighting disbelief. "And when will the visit take place?"

"Tomorrow morning at nine o'clock," came the reply.

The next morning, everyone rose early to prepare for the visit. At 9 a.m., Piero and the senior staff gathered at the gate to welcome the president. There was no sign of him. They waited and waited. It wasn't until the early afternoon that a long black car drew up at the hospital gates. As Idi Amin stepped from his car, a team of hefty bodyguards surrounded him and never left his side.

Piero and Lucille moved forward to greet the president, and then they led him on a tour of the hospital. After the visit, they served him a cup of tea. Idi Amin was an imposing man, much larger than his photos suggested. He lavishly praised the hospital, especially remarking on the cleanliness. And before he left, he said, "I see that you have a very strong sense of discipline here. I wish I had such discipline in my own army." Then he stood up, said "Thank you" to everyone, and was gone.

∞

Idi Amin's reign of terror lasted for eight years, from 1971 to 1979. The carnage that swept Uganda during that period was almost impossible for outsiders to comprehend. By the late 1970s, the country's infrastructure had been virtually wiped out. The economy had collapsed and most hospitals and health clinics had closed. Roads were cracked and riddled with potholes, cities were turned into garbage dumps, and utilities had completely fallen apart.

Because of the chaos, authorities suspended all flights into Kampala and closed all borders. This meant that foreigners could no longer visit the country, so the once lucrative tourism industry dried up. In any case, there was little left for tourists to enjoy since soldiers had killed most of the country's wild animals for meat and ivory. The land once known throughout the world as "the pearl of Africa" lay in shreds.

Many Ugandans despaired of their future. As they looked around at the widespread devastation, they wondered how their country could ever recover.

There was one small glimmer of hope on the horizon. On April 11, 1979 – eight years after the celebrations that marked Idi Amin's rise to power – an army of soldiers from neighbouring Tanzania, together with a handful of Ugandan exiles, pushed their way into Kampala, stormed Amin's compound, and managed to overthrow the despot. Amin fled north to Libya, and then to Saudi Arabia, where he remained until his death in 2002.

Ugandans everywhere celebrated Amin's departure with dancing and the beating of drums. In

Kampala, people swarmed around the steps of Parliament House. They prayed for those who died at the hands of Idi Amin. They also prayed for peace.

The euphoria that spread across the country was short-lived. The Tanzanian army that had come to save Uganda now seemed intent on ravaging it. After they ousted Amin, they overran Kampala, and in the weeks that followed, the country exploded into civil war. Two successive governments tried to restore order but failed. Milton Obote returned from exile and was elected president for the second time, but he was unable to bring about calm.

As the civil war escalated, killing and looting spread, food supplies dwindled, and hospitals ran out of medicine. Emergency rations of food and drugs poured into Uganda but were never enough.

The northern region was hit particularly hard. People there were facing serious drought and famine, telephones and postal service had collapsed, and road-blocks prevented any traffic and supplies from getting through. Almost overnight, Lacor Hospital found itself completely cut off from the rest of the country.

Worst of all, the whole of the north was now over-run by soldiers. Many of them were deserters from Amin's army while others were bandits who moved around in groups, shooting, stealing, and looting all the government buildings. In Gulu, they ransacked the post office, the hospital, the bank, and the police sta-tion. They even stormed the prisons and set all the prisoners free. "Most of the people are now in hiding or living in the bush," Lucille wrote to her sister. "Gulu is completely deserted and devastated. We realized it was a ghost city when we finally reached the government hospital and found that all the doctors had left long before."

As a result of so much unrest, many of the remaining foreigners fled the country. Lucille and Piero stayed, as always. Thanks to them, Lacor Hospital was the only building in the region still functioning, though sadly they felt obliged to close the Health Centres. Wounded soldiers and civilians from both sides of the conflict came to the hospital from miles around to seek medical care. No one was refused treatment.

Once again, Lucille became a war surgeon. She worked around the clock, operating on the never-ending stream of wounded soldiers who arrived at their door. When the electricity failed, she relied on a small emergency generator that provided a flickering light and barely enough power to keep fridges running and drugs cool. By nightfall, she and Piero would return home exhausted. They would sink into their comfy couch, light a pair of candles, and then switch on the shortwave radio for the latest BBC newscast, their one link to the outside world.

∞

Lucille and Piero were only too aware that they were in a region where fighting erupted almost daily. Nevertheless, they always felt they were safe in the confines of the hospital compound. That was about to change.

On 14 May 1979, their sense of security ended abruptly on what Lucille later called "our day of terror."

Around noon a bus full of soldiers stopped outside the compound. Lucille had just begun a delicate abdominal operation on a wounded soldier, when suddenly the electricity failed and she heard gunshots outside. No sooner had she managed to activate the generator and return to her patient than a noisy gang of thirty armed men stormed through the gates and into the hospital. Most of the nurses fled in fear. A couple remained and helped Lucille rush through the wards and shove the patients under the beds for protection.

The rebels dashed across the compound, shooting at the sky, while their leaders barked out orders demanding that hospital officials hand over all their petrol supplies. Piero arrived on the scene and flatly refused to comply with their demands. Disgruntled, they left empty-handed. The compound fell silent.

The silence did not last for long. At 6 p.m. the same thugs returned, and the real terror began. Twelve cars full of soldiers, deserters, and members of their families stopped in front of the hospital. Piero went to meet them outside the gate. They fired their guns into the sky, demanded entry into the hospital, and asked again for their petrol supplies. Piero agreed to hand over some petrol but insisted they leave their rifles outside the gate. This annoyed their leader, who immediately seized Piero, thumped him on the right ear, and kicked him in the legs.

Piero tried to flee. The irate leader grabbed a rifle from his car and fired a stream of bullets, missing Piero by a hair's breadth. Terrified, Piero managed to reach the gatekeeper's hut and lock himself in, where he sat, cowering. The gunman stood outside, rifle at the ready.

Ten minutes ticked by... Suddenly, a woman jumped from the car. "Stop stop! Do not kill our doctor." The gunman looked startled. The woman, who had just realized what was going on, was his mother. She had been a patient of Lucille's.

"Do not kill our doctor," she pleaded again. He put down his weapon, walked slowly to his car, got in, and drove away.

∞

By 7 p.m., all was quiet again – but only for a moment. As Lucille and Piero were walking back to their house, they encountered an old woman who had staggered into the compound looking for Lucille. The soldiers who had just driven away had broken into her house nearby and demanded that she hand over all her money. She had only ten Ugandan shillings, which so infuriated the thugs that they shot her three times.

The woman could barely walk. Lucille helped carry her over to the operating theatre, donned a surgical gown and gloves, and worked until after 11 p.m. treating the woman's wounds. She managed to save her life.

Near midnight, Lucille returned home. As she stepped through her front door, she saw that while she had been operating on the wounded woman, the house had been broken into and ransacked. Some of the same thugs had turned out drawers and cupboards and made off with the reserve petrol supply. They had taken all the drugs they could find and most of Lucille's surgical equipment. They also had stolen the couple's shortwave radio, their record player, and nearly all their shoes!

The next morning, Lucille and Piero learned that one of their trucks, three ambulances, and two cars were gone. One of the cars belonged to Piero, but because he had prudently removed the carburetor, the thieves had been unable to get beyond the gate of the hospital compound.

Luckily, everyone within the compound was alive and unhurt. The only casualty was Piero, who had suffered a punctured eardrum from the thump on the head and later required surgery to repair it.

⚬

The following days were quiet, but everyone felt nervous and fearful that the soldiers would return at any moment. Most of the staff had left, which meant that the few who remained had to work doubly hard to deal with the increasing number of patients. Lacor was now the only hospital in the whole country that remained open, and wounded soldiers seeking treatment were arriving from all across Uganda.

When things finally began to ease up, Lucille found herself pondering her future. *What shall we do? How can we go on living and working under such circumstances?* She thought about the local people whom she had come to love and respect. *I feel so much a part of their life, but how long can we continue to help them?* Dominique was still at school in Kenya, so their links to Africa were doubly strong.

She shared her thoughts in a letter to her sisters. "I know for the moment that we have no choice. We are the only doctors in the whole region so we must stay. But after that?

"We don't think we are in any state – mentally or physically – to carry out any future projects. I guess we have to wait and see what happens... For now, we would like to take a long holiday this summer with Dominique. We haven't seen her since January and we have had no news from her for two months."

∞

Late in 1979 Lucille and Piero finally managed to leave for a few weeks' holiday in Italy, where Dominique joined them. They returned to Uganda much refreshed. In a letter to her friends at Christmas, Lucille expressed her hopes and concerns for the future.

"Uganda is beginning to emerge from the dark ages and is starting the long journey of reconstruction... We returned from Italy and found the hospital and our house all newly painted – thanks to the wonderful sisters – and our nurses and student nurses all welcomed us back enthusiastically. It was good to be home.

"Back too came all the children with their various ailments – anemia, malnutrition, malaria – very often arriving much too late to be helped. There are no more bullet wounds just now but so many chronic patients who had stopped their treatment because of the war...

"Now that everybody is back in Lacor, we are hoping to organize many new medical services. One of the doctors has already restored the programme of Health

Education... We are planning to reopen the three Health Centres within the next year. We expect to receive funds from Italy to build a new cancer and TB ward, Brother Toni Biasin is installing the new radio-therapy equipment, and John, our Jack-of-all-trades, is now becoming an expert in making calipers from old children's shoes and pieces of rod and wood... Piero has even started again to talk about his old dream of a Farm School for handicapped children. And why not?

"Thank God that, after eighteen years in Gulu, we still do not feel too old to dream."

8

A Devastating Blow

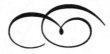

That was Guido on the phone. He has received the results of the tests. Piero, negative. Lucille, positive.

– Piero Corti, August 1985

As the 1980s unfolded, Lucille and Piero were both deeply absorbed in getting things at Lacor running again. Although it was now relatively peaceful in the north, the civil war dragged on and left everyone with a feeling of uncertainty. For the first time, Piero admitted to being uneasy about the situation, but he dismissed the thought of ever leaving. "As a religious man, I am convinced that we should stay in Uganda," he told Lucille. "I am certain that God has directed us to

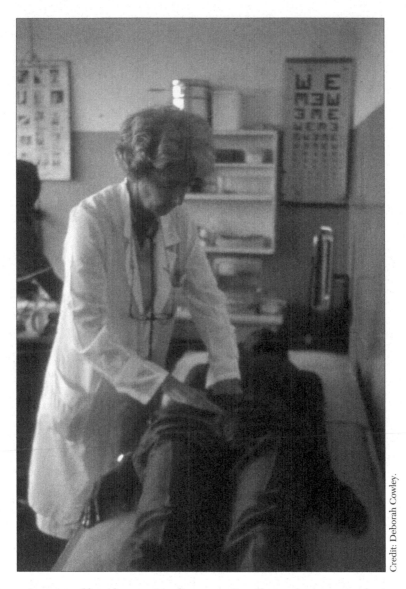

In spite of her devastating diagnosis, Lucille continues to work.

remain at the hospital and to help where we are so desperately needed." Lucille nodded. "Do you remember my dream, Lucille? There is still so much to be done to turn this hospital into a world-class facility."

In spite of the unsettled state of the country, Piero decided to go ahead with a serious campaign of expansion. He wrote hundreds of letters and badgered friends and family, governments, and non-governmental organizations for help. He flew to Italy to arrange for a huge shipment of equipment and medicines. Much to everyone's surprise, he achieved what had seemed impossible. Even though manpower and materials were difficult to find, by the mid-1980s he had managed to build a new seventy-bed unit for medical patients and a shelter for parents and families of the sick where they could live while caring for the patient. He also created a ninety-bed children's ward, a fifty-one-bed ward for obstetric and gynecology patients, and a sixty-six-bed ward for surgery patients.

The new facilities came none too soon. During that period, there was an epidemic of measles and a dramatic increase in cases of pneumonia and dehydration, particularly among children. There was also a rise in the number of tuberculosis cases – more than twenty new admissions each month – so Piero built a thirty-six-bed ward for TB patients. He later added an outpatient clinic for those with eye diseases and a thirty-six-bed ward for cancer patients. He also managed to secure equipment for all the new facilities.

Piero then used his persuasive skills to raise funds for a radiology department with three X-ray machines and radiation equipment for the treatment of cancer patients. As a result, the hospital became an important referral centre for patients with cancer, who came from all over Uganda for chemotherapy and radiation treatments.

Of all the projects Piero managed to complete, one stood out as his real pride and joy: a pair of handsome new operating theatres that he offered as a special gift to Lucille.

෴

The smart new facilities gave everyone a boost. They could now accept more patients and offer many more services. However, in spite of all the new furnishings, the staff found they were often missing some small but critical piece of equipment. One day, a mother brought her three-year-old boy to the hospital with a case of hydrocephalus, an excess of fluid on the brain. If the child wasn't treated immediately, there could be serious brain damage, and he would probably live his life in a vegetative state. Without treatment, he might even die. Lucille checked the boy carefully and found that, in order to treat him, she would need to insert a special valve that would drain the fluid from the brain. There was no such valve anywhere in Uganda.

Even when Piero was juggling many different jobs, he would go to any lengths to help an especially needy case. The minute he heard about the child's condition, he sent an urgent radio message explaining the situation to Dr. Arshad Warley, a good friend in London. Warley jumped into action. He called a neurosurgeon who readily supplied the required valve and packed it up with detailed instructions on how to insert it. By good fortune, Warley was travelling that same week to his native South Africa. He stopped off in Uganda to personally hand over the precious package to Piero.

When Lucille received the valve, she immediately scanned the notes and set to work. She had never performed such an operation before, but with the directions propped up in front of her, she worked steadily for four hours and managed to insert the valve and save the child. Impressed, Warley said: "That was a very difficult operation for someone to undertake in a big city hospital. To do it up there in the bush was truly remarkable."

A beaming Piero added: "Just give Lucille the instructions and she can do anything, absolutely anything."

∞

Dominique had by now left her school in Kenya and returned to Italy where she had enrolled at the University of Milan for a course in foreign languages. On one of her visits home, she was sitting with her mother on the veranda of their bungalow, talking about her life at the university and about her studies. Quite suddenly, she announced: "Guess what, Mama... I've decided I would like to study medicine!"

Lucille was thrilled with Dominique's decision to change faculties. Imagine her own daughter wanting to be a doctor! This was a dream come true. When Piero heard the news, he too was elated. "Does this mean you will give up your riding?" he asked.

"Oh no. I'm already preparing for a big championship in Lombardy."

When the school year began, Dominique, then twenty-two, enrolled in the University of Milan's Faculty of Medicine. It was the same school from which Piero had graduated over thirty years before.

∞

In the early 1980s, as the unrest in Uganda continued, few people were aware that a devastating and even more deadly enemy was now stalking the land. The enemy was a previously unknown disease that at first appeared to affect only men, usually young men. They turned up at clinics with serious weight loss, a high fever, a persistent cough, and chronic diarrhea that often lasted several months. Then women too began arriving with the same symptoms. Lucille was as puzzled as others about this strange new disease. She tried using antibiotics that normally helped relieve these various symptoms, but they had no effect.

Lucille and others eventually discovered that these were the first ominous signs of the virus the world would come to know as HIV – human immunodeficiency virus – which very often leads to the condition known as AIDS.

Researchers learned that HIV is carried in the blood and transmitted either sexually or through transfusions of infected blood. The virus weakens the immune system so that anyone carrying it easily picks up other infections. Probably the disease had been brought into Uganda by truck drivers crossing into the country from neighbouring Kenya or by the Tanzanian soldiers who had overrun Uganda after the departure of Idi Amin.

The first hazy reports of the disease began to circulate in Uganda around 1982. Before long, health professionals found themselves dealing with a highly contagious disease the Ugandans called "slim" because of the skeletal appearance of the victims in the last stages. Little did they know then that it would soon become an epidemic that would claim the lives of more than a million of their countrymen – one-twentieth of the population.

The unexpected arrival of AIDS meant an ever-increasing workload for the hospital staff at Lacor. Lucille was now seeing well over two hundred people a day in the outpatient clinic as well as doing many emergency operations beyond the routine ones. Luckily, she seemed to have unlimited energy and appeared to be undaunted by the extra workload. Her friend, Canadian pediatrician Dr. Elizabeth Hillman, who was a frequent visitor to Lacor, said: "Lucille always had the most tremendous amount of energy. She would work until she was limp and exhausted. If there was an emergency, she would think nothing of working through the night."

Lucille did not deny that she was blessed with an abundance of energy and that she had a compulsion to work flat out, often for many hours without a break. Luckily, there were now two younger doctors who could help with minor surgery, but she was still the only one who could undertake the more complicated cases – and there were at least five or six of those every week.

Piero and Lucille were also beginning to receive help from medical interns from Makerere University who were sent to Lacor for training. One of these was a young medical student, Matthew Lukwiya. Matthew turned out to be a bright and dedicated doctor, especially gifted with children, and he quickly became one of Lucille's most stalwart helpers. To Lucille and Piero's delight, Matthew later chose to return to Lacor, where he became an important and loyal presence in the hospital.

∞

During this same period Lucille began to notice that she was tiring easily and needed to rest more often. She passed her fatigue off as a question of age. She had recently turned fifty-six and could not expect to have the same energy level as a twenty-year-old. She contracted malaria, and for several weeks her temperature hovered around 40 degrees. She was also plagued by a persistent cough that dragged on for almost a month. Piero suspected chronic bronchitis and arranged to have her lungs X-rayed. They found nothing abnormal.

As the months progressed, Lucille grew angry with herself and annoyed by her decreasing energy. When she could not keep to her usual busy routine, she became depressed.

In April 1985 Lucille and Piero had just returned from a short Easter holiday when Lucille became aware of a severe pain in her left shoulder. Gradually, the pain spread throughout the shoulder, then to her upper body and down into her arms. Piero concluded that she had shingles, a virus similar to chicken pox that affects sensitive nerves and causes intense pain. The pain lasted for several weeks.

Lucille was particularly alarmed by the fact that she was losing weight. She had always weighed around forty-eight kilos, but now she had dropped to forty-four. Deep down, she began to wonder if there was something seriously wrong with her.

That summer, Lucille and Piero decided to visit Canada to see Lucille's father, who was seriously ill. She had not been home when her mother had died eleven years before so it was important for her to see her father while he was still alive. They stopped first in Milan to pick up Dominique, and while they were there, both Lucille and Piero arranged to have some tests. Lucille had found a few tiny lumps under her jaw and under her armpits, so specialists checked her lymph glands for cancer. The results were negative. They also took a series of blood tests and promised to phone the results to her in Canada.

The three flew on to Montreal. On the plane, Piero grew increasingly worried by Lucille's condition and began to think of all the possible scenarios. What if the disease was fatal and Lucille died before he did? Throughout their adult life, the two had been inseparable. Lucille had been his constant companion for almost twenty-five years, and he could not imagine how he could possibly live without her.

In Montreal, they joined Lucille's sisters, Monique and Yolande, at their parents' cottage outside Montreal. Lucille had a happy reunion with her father, her sisters, and many nieces and nephews who gathered in one of her favourite corners of Quebec.

One morning, as the family sat together relaxing by the pool, the phone rang. Monique went inside to answer it. The voice on the line said that the call was from Italy. Monique passed the phone to Piero. He listened silently, and then he hung up. For several minutes he sat by the phone with his head in his hands. Then he got up and walked slowly out to the pool where Lucille was sitting with her sisters.

He sat down beside Lucille, took her hand in his, and said: "That was Guido on the phone." His voice cracked as he said, in barely a whisper. "He has received the results of the tests." He paused, then added four words: "Piero, negative. Lucille, positive."

The tests showed that Dr. Lucille, the woman who had treated hundreds of AIDS patients, had herself become a victim of the disease.

Lucille was stunned. In one sense, she was relieved to know at last the reason for all her recent health problems: the cough, the recurring pneumonia, fever, and weight loss. But it took some time to sink in that she – the one who had always felt invincible and fearless about contracting any disease – had now joined the legions of people with AIDS.

The family was devastated by the news. They all kept saying to each other "Why does someone who helps so many people deserve such a thing? It just doesn't seem fair."

Later, as Lucille sat alone with Piero, she found herself wondering how she could have contracted AIDS. As she looked back, she realized that many of the hundreds of soldiers she had operated on were undoubtedly carrying the disease. She recalled the number of times she had repaired gunshot wounds inflicted by soft bullets and how she had probed into the soldiers' flesh with her fingers. She remembered being stabbed by sharp fragments of bone, which had ripped open her gloves and pricked her fingers. At that time, neither she nor anyone could have known that some of her patients were carrying this deadly and highly contagious disease.

As they sat by the pool in Quebec, Lucille put on a brave face. From the beginning of her medical career, she had always taken for granted what she called 'the risks of the job.' But when she spoke of risks, she had thought about diseases that could easily be cured by antibiotics. She had never thought in terms of a fatal disease such as AIDS, a disease for which there was no cure.

In spite of the news they received, the holiday in Canada was a positive experience for Lucille. She enjoyed being with her sisters and seeing old friends again. She shared many special moments with her father. She loved the cottage life, where she ate well, put on some weight, and looked better than she had when she arrived.

∞

On their way home to Uganda, Piero and Lucille stopped in London to consult Dr. Anthony Pinching, a world-renowned specialist in immunology and AIDS. Lucille told him she wanted to know her prognosis; she wanted to know the truth. She described the long list of symptoms that had plagued her over the past few years. Then Dr. Pinching spoke: "Since you asked for the truth, I can tell you that at the stage you are, I believe there is a 25 per cent chance that you will live for two years. But then," he added, "I could always be wrong."

Lucille was visibly shaken. That meant she had one chance in four of living beyond 1987 and dying from any number of minor illnesses. "Oh well," she said stoically. "I must just learn to fight each illness I get, as best I can, one illness at a time."

Anthony Pinching was able to reassure her about her medical work. "Do not think that you will catch all the germs of all your patients," he said. "But you must be very careful, especially with tuberculosis patients. TB is a highly contagious disease. You can certainly continue to work with your outpatients but you must always be very careful."

There was one question she had not dared to ask. Could she continue to practise surgery without threatening the health of her patients? After all, surgery was her life and it was in the operating room that she felt most useful.

On her return to Uganda, Lucille consulted a friend and colleague, Wilson Carswell. He was a surgeon at Mulago Hospital in Kampala. "If the condition of the patient is not life-threatening or if the operation can be carried out by another doctor, you should not operate. If, however, the condition is life-threatening, and if you are the only one who can carry out the operation, you should go ahead. But do so with the utmost care."

Lucille was greatly relieved. She returned to work with renewed vigour. In the mornings, she continued

to see her outpatients. She passed the routine operations on to other surgeons but continued to perform
the more complicated ones herself. Her work was her
life. She was determined to continue helping those in
need, as long as her health permitted.

UGANDA PEOPLE DEMOCRATIC ARMY
UGANDA PEOPLE DEMOCRATIC MOVEMENT

To DR. CORTI Lacor hospital
From Operation Commander
CRACK-DOWN BATTALIAN 115 BDE

Be informed that, We have your
nursing staff by the name NWAZI AMOTI
She has been our enemy number
one for along time. But now we have
got her to be Politicised and trained
to work Under our movement

PLEASE DON'T TRY TO BRING
ANY GOVERNMENT TROOPS TO Look
FOR HER. IF YOU DO, SHE WILL
DIE AUTOMATICALLY

We hope we are clear and Precise
follow our order, and she will be safe
up to Kampala.   OPTO.
                              CPT. 1-U-37
             Thanks OPIO

                  CPT OKWERA

Note sent from a Commander of the UPDA concerning
the kidnapping of a young nurse who worked at the hospital.

9

More Challenges

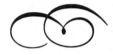

Lucille is always the first to remind me that we are not here on a two or three year contract but for our whole life. Her sense of duty borders on heroism...
— Piero Corti to his brother Eugenio, January 1986

When Piero and Lucille returned to Uganda in the fall of 1985, they were both still struggling to come to terms with the reality of Lucille's disease. It was a crushing blow to them both. Typically, Lucille was remarkably accepting and philosophical, while Piero was visibly shattered.

"From the start, Lucille has been magnificent," he wrote to his brother Corrado in December 1985. "She has not changed her behaviour at all, except that she is a little quieter than she was... Because of her illness, we are living much more intensely than before... However, I am very, very distressed... and I need your prayers."

Nothing, not even the confirmation of such a debilitating and hopeless illness, would stop Lucille from continuing her work. She did agree to reduce her workload a little by spending only three days a week in the operating theatre. This was only because she had contracted dermatitis, an eczema-like rash on her hands, and it flared up when she wore rubber gloves.

Luckily, there were now other surgeons who could help out. Some were Italian doctors sent by the Italian Ministry of Foreign Affairs. More and more were Africans, graduates from Makerere University in Kampala, many of whom had trained under Lucille and could do the routine operations. And there was Matthew Lukwiya, another Makerere graduate, who had already worked as an intern at the hospital. He had chosen to return to Lacor as a fully qualified doctor, and no one was happier about this than Lucille and Piero. They considered him to be one of best of the young doctors they had trained and one whom they felt might someday take over their work.

Lucille may have cut down her time in the operating room but she did not reduce the long hours she spent dealing with the ever-increasing influx of outpatients. There were now more than two hundred people a day lined up outside her office, awaiting help. She saw them all, greeted each one in Acholi, which she now spoke well, and checked them over carefully.

She also spent much of her time and energy helping to train a steady stream of Ugandan medical interns
from Makerere University. Since 1982, Lacor Hospital
had been recognized by the government as a teaching
hospital, and training had become an important priority for both Lucille and Piero. "The training those
young interns received at Lacor was just fantastic," said
Sally Fagan-Wyse, then UNICEF representative in
Kampala. "The Cortis set the highest possible standards and were both such inspiring examples for those
students."

Lucille and Piero had always hoped that one day,
the hospital would be run and staffed entirely by
Africans. At last, they were beginning to make impressive strides in that direction.

∽

In January 1986, fifteen years after the coup that
brought Idi Amin to power, the forces of a young guerrilla leader, Yoweri Museveni, staged another coup. At
first, Museveni appeared to bring renewed hope to the
country, and there was an uneasy peace. But that hope
was soon shattered by the emergence of several rebel
groups who were determined to challenge the new
government. As these groups proliferated, insecurity
spread and travel once more became dangerous.

To compound the already precarious situation,
refugees from civil wars in neighbouring Sudan and
Rwanda were crowding into Uganda. This influx of
refugees placed even more stress on the country's
already fragile infrastructure.

Piero's family in Italy and the couple's many friends around the world grew increasingly worried about them and wrote letters begging them to leave Lacor and enjoy a quiet retirement elsewhere. At night, in the quiet of their house, Piero and Lucille would read and re-read these letters and try to contemplate the possibility of leaving Lacor. "Everyone we know thinks we should pack up and leave," said Lucille, fingering the most recent packet of letters. "Do you think we should leave, Piero?"

"Definitely not," replied Piero without hesitation. He cast a reassuring glance at Lucille. That same night, he wrote to his brother Eugenio, who had also expressed his concern: "Do you really think we can leave the hospital and abandon everyone here?" Piero asked. "I would only leave if Lucille wants me to do so. But she is always the first to remind me that, when we came here, it was not with a two or three year contract. It was for our whole life. Her sense of duty borders on heroism... She continues to demand the impossible of herself, even when her health is not what it was."

So they stayed. That spring, they were rewarded by one piece of good news that shone brightly upon the dreary landscape: the World Health Organization had named Lucille and Piero winners of their prestigious $100,000 Sasakawa Prize. The committee gave special praise to their initiatives in the field of primary health care – training health care workers so they could help fight malnutrition and run vaccination clinics in the three health units they had set up in the surrounding countryside.

The Sasakawa Prize was a fitting tribute to twenty-five years of service. The couple travelled to Geneva in May 1986 to receive the prize before a large assembly of Ministers of Health from around the world.

They returned to Uganda to find the country deteriorating once again into chaos. Rebel activity was on the rise, especially in the north where the hospital was located, and this spread fear around the whole region. The postal system had collapsed again and there were more electricity cuts. For almost a month during the autumn they were without power and had to pay exorbitant prices for diesel fuel to keep their own generators running for eight to ten hours a day. "Luckily one of the Brothers managed to install a solar panel on the roof of our house," Lucille told Lise. "That way, we could recharge our batteries and get some very dim light when the electricity and generators stopped functioning."

She wrote again, as the year was drawing to a close: "The situation is now so sad and very depressing. Every evening, we can hear the sound of machine-gun fire. A few weeks ago, the rebels hurled two bombs into the little market in front of the hospital. There were two dead and thirty wounded, all women and children."

As Christmas approached, there appeared to be little cause for celebration.

"This time it is not the war that is the problem," Lucille wrote to Lise just before Christmas. "This time, it is the guerrillas. The hospital is caught between two rival groups – the NRA (the National Resistance Army) of President Museveni and the rebels who call themselves the Uganda People's Democratic Army (the UPDA). During the day we get some protection by the NRA. But at night when they go back to Gulu, the others arrive. So far, neither of them seems to want to confront us but almost every night, we can hear the sounds of gunfire and bombs exploding on the road across just across from us."

Very few patients were coming to the hospital because everyone was afraid to travel. Most of their staff, also afraid, had left. "I am the only surgeon here right now," Lucille said in another letter to Lise. "My assistant is on holiday and the woman gynecologist has said that she can no longer work under such tense conditions so she has gone too. Our new surgeon, who should have begun his two-year contract in September, has still not arrived because of the situation." Once again, the Cortis were virtually alone.

The next year, 1987, looked even more ominous. Opposition to the new president was growing, most seriously in the north, and with it emerged another group of rebels calling itself the "Lord's Resistance Army" (the LRA). This merciless group adopted a new and terrifying weapon: they not only carried out indiscriminate killings but also kidnapped children and used them to help fight their war. In a few short months, they captured more than 11,000 children and teenagers.

The LRA also became known for its widespread rape of women, and Lacor Hospital was one of their targets. One night in January, an armed soldier broke into the dormitory where relatives of the patients were sleeping and opened fire. He then looked over all the women and fixed on one of them, the mother of a sick child. He ordered her to undress and raped her in full view of all the others.

Lucille and Piero were horrified. They had asked the government for better security but it had still not been provided. Things were becoming tense and fear was running so high that, after much deliberating, they believed that the only course open to them was to close down part of the hospital.

They discharged some of the patients and moved others to the more secure hospital in Gulu. This left only half the beds in the surgery ward still occupied. The maternity ward and the cancer ward were both empty because the train that brought patients to the hospital from all over the country was no longer running. Also, to their great sadness, Piero felt obliged to close the three outlying health clinics that had proven to be such admirable models for primary health care since 1979 and that had helped them win the Sasakawa Prize the previous year.

Although the number of patients had been reduced, the hospital was by no means empty. Civil wars still raged in Rwanda and in the Sudan, so more and more refugees from these countries crossed into northern Uganda. For many, Lacor Hospital became their safe haven. At one point, the cancer ward sheltered almost four hundred women and children. Hundreds more slept on the verandas and in the grounds of the hospital.

∽

The two rebel groups, the LRA and the UPDA, continued their menacing tactics. Travel to and from Kampala became increasingly dangerous, and anyone venturing on such a journey needed to join a military convoy in order to avoid ambush. The atmosphere was tense. Everyone in the hospital feared that an attack was imminent.

Few were surprised when, on the night of 31 March 1987, four rebels of the UPDA broke into the hospital, firing their guns into the air. They said they were searching for Amooti Mwazi, a young nurse who belonged to the Bunyoros tribe from the south. "She is a spy for the government," they bellowed. "We are here to kidnap her." At the sound of the commotion, Lucille and Piero dashed over to the dormitory to try and reason with the group.

"You cannot take this woman," Lucille shouted.

"Yes we can," they answered. "She is a spy."

"She is not," replied Lucille. "She is a nurse who looks after the sick, your sick people, and all the Acholis."

The insurgents brushed past Lucille and seized the young woman. Lucille begged them to spare the young nurse's life, even to take her instead. They ignored her pleas. Piero tried to stop them and they answered with a burst of gunfire over his head. Before their very eyes, they carried Amooti away.

Piero was so distraught by the incident that the following day, he decided to close the rest of the hospital to all except emergency cases. He sent out a notice saying that it would remain closed until their nurse was safely returned.

Two days later, Piero received a letter signed by the "Operations Commander" of the UPDA "Crack-Down Battalion," which confirmed that they were holding Amooti. "Be informed that we have your nursing staff by the name of Mwazi Amooti," it read. "She has been our enemy number one for a long time. But now we have got her to be politicized and trained to work under our movement." It added, "Do not try to bring any government troops to look for her. If you do, she will die."

The Commander had attached a short, handwritten letter to Dr. Corti from Amooti. It read:

Excuse me Dr. – this is to inform you that I'm still alive but don't make any mistake of going to the NRA soldiers to come and try to rescue me. I'm asked to stay behind and serve as a nurse. So, if you really treasure my life give whoever brings this letter to you some drugs, i.e. antibiotics, chloroquine, aspirin, some syringes and needles, gauzes.

Yours faithfully,
Mwazi B. Amooti.

Piero received a second message from the UPDA Commander a few days later. It said that, in fact, the group had made a mistake: they had captured the wrong woman. Amooti was not the spy they had thought she was and they were now prepared to release her.

Lucille and Piero received a message telling them to go and pick up Amooti at a designated place seven kilometres from the hospital. When they got to the spot, they found Amooti but were horrified to discover that she had been severely tortured during her captivity. She had been burned on her legs, across her back and under her breasts. "They just wanted to make her admit that she was a spy," Lucille explained in a letter to her sister. "After this event, you can imagine the panic and fear that spread among our staff."

∞

That one incident may have ended, but it was not the last. On Monday 19 April, another group of rebels from the LRA burst into the hospital compound, yelping and waving rifles. Lucille was reading in her living room when about fifteen members of the gang marched over to her house, broke down the door, and stormed inside. They were all carrying rifles and they threatened both Lucille and Piero. Moving through the house, they turned out all the drawers and stuffed everything they could find into sacks. Then, as abruptly as they came, they left.

Everything happened so quickly. The generator was off, so the place was in the dark, and when Lucille got up to check the damage, she tripped, fell, and injured her thigh. "This was a real nuisance and soon developed into myositis [an inflammation of the muscle]. It was very, very painful," she wrote.

Piero's concern for Lucille grew when an ultrasound showed that the infection in her thigh was spreading to her pelvis. If it spread farther, it could become extremely serious. Her intense pain was also increasing daily, so Piero decided to take no chances and arranged to fly Lucille to London for treatment.

In London, their friend Arshad Warley met them at the airport. Warley could see immediately that Lucille was in pain, and he felt deeply saddened. In spite of her pain, Lucille said she had always wanted to see Cambridge, one of the most picturesque English towns, so Warley and his wife drove them there for a short visit. Lucille was thrilled to have the chance to gaze upon the centuries-old King's College chapel and to sit on the river's edge watching the students pole their way in punts along the river.

They were walking back to their car through the town when Piero grabbed Warley's arm and whispered: "Arshad, I am afraid we are going to lose Lucille."

"Remember that Lucille is very strong," Warley reassured him.

They drove to the London hospital, where Anthony Pinching was waiting for them. Eighteen months had passed since Lucille's previous visit, and she had not forgotten that the same doctor had told her that she had only a 25 per cent chance of surviving more than two years. He treated her at once with a strong dose of antibiotics. After a few days' rest, she had regained her strength and announced that she was ready to return home to Uganda.

They arrived back in Gulu to find that conditions were not much better. "Life is still very difficult here," Lucille wrote to her sister Lise in late April. "There has been no electricity for almost three months. No trains are running but worst of all, we seem to find ourselves in a sort of 'no man's land.' The government troops (the NRA) stay in Gulu while the guerrillas (the UPDA) roam around just north of the hospital so we are at the mercy of these hooligans. We cannot call the police (who practically do not exist around here anyway) and the army refuses to come and give us any protection.

"Once again, we are practically cut off from the rest of the country. The road is unsafe except for a military convoy. The postal service is no longer running so we must rely on a few relief planes to send out our letters."

The dangerous conditions that existed throughout the region took a heavy toll on the remaining hospital staff. "Already, since 15 February, we have lost two interns and one doctor," Lucille wrote. "Today, three interns and one more doctor have left, as well as my assistant in surgery. Another doctor will also leave as soon as he has taught Piero and one of the African doctors how to operate the recently donated dialysis machine.

"All this is very, very sad," she continued. "After twenty-six years we were so close to our aim of building a medical complex which was to become one of the best in Uganda and also one that was completely Africanized. We had some really outstanding Ugandan doctors and we were also innovating in many fields: we had the first radiotherapy service in all Uganda and were soon to have cobalt therapy as well; we had the first ultrasound service; and our very successful programme of primary health care was up and running again." She was fighting back tears as she wrote. "It is all so sad. That is all I can say."

∞

The year 1987 turned out to be the toughest yet for Lucille and Piero. Not only did political events manage to curtail most of their hospital activities but also as the year progressed, Lucille's health began to deteriorate. She no longer enjoyed eating and had little appetite. Piero would sit by her side and encourage her to eat. "Just try one bite," he would say, offering her a spoonful of food. He had little success.

Lucille also began to be plagued by illness. She had frequent bouts of pneumonia and recurring malaria. Even the smallest accident that once she would have ignored now turned into a major crisis.

One day, Lucille accidentally tripped over the leg of her bed and injured her groin. The injury led to a high fever, then an abscess developed, which meant there was an infection in the tissue. It became so serious that Piero felt they should operate. But the only surgeon who could perform such an operation had left the hospital. Piero decided that, for the first time in his life, he would operate on his own wife.

He gave Lucille an epidural anesthetic. When she was completely numb, he proceeded to cut and drain the abscess.

The operation went well, but the pain and fever increased. Piero feared there might be a secondary infection and a further operation would be much more complicated and beyond his ability. He saw no other solution but to arrange for another visit to London.

Once again, Arshad Warley met them at the airport. He was dismayed to see how weak Lucille had become since her last visit a few months before. As he drove the couple across London to St. Mary's Hospital, he wondered how much longer Lucille could possibly live. *She is very, very ill*, he thought. *I honestly think she is going to die very soon.*

Anthony Pinching was waiting for them at the hospital and confirmed that the high fever was a direct result of the abscess. He also said it was the presence of the HIV virus that was preventing it from healing. He put her on antibiotics at once.

Lucille recovered in record time. No one was more surprised than Arshad Warley. "She rallied and regained her strength quicker than anyone would have thought possible. It was absolutely amazing." After three weeks of convalescence, Lucille was up and ready to fly back to Uganda.

10

Losing Hope

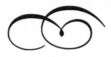

> *How can you live for three years among all this misery and violence?... We are losing hope and without hope, life is no longer life... We have never been so close to abandoning everything here.*
> – Piero to his brother Corrado, 14 Feb 1989

Lucille and Piero arrived back in Gulu in the autumn of 1987 to find that little had changed. There would be periods of calm, and then the rebels would appear again and disrupt the whole region. The unsettled conditions caused much hardship: the staff continued to be so fearful of attacks and kidnapping that they would pack up and leave. Because transportation was still

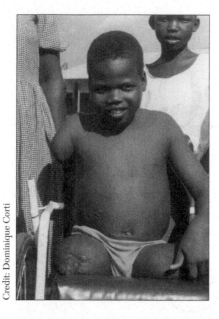

Young boy who accidentally stepped on a land mine. His legs and right arm could not be salvaged, and he now lives in an orphanage near the hospital because life in a rural village would be impossible for him.

Credit: Dominique Corti

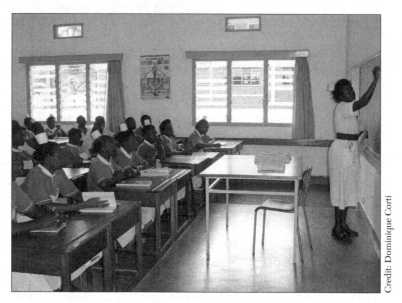

Credit: Dominique Corti

Classroom in the Lacor Nursing Training School.
Lessons are carried out in the classes, but students start working
in the hospital right from the first year.

sporadic, the sick could not travel to the hospital. Only about forty patients a day were arriving for consultation – even when a new epidemic of measles had broken out and AIDS continued to take its devastating toll.

Lucille had relatively little work to do and she became frustrated by the inactivity. She missed her heavy workload and the satisfaction she received from helping her patients. The presence of her disease had given her a new sense of urgency. She felt her time was limited, and she was anxious to do as much as possible while she could.

With so little work, she had more time to think. She began to see herself as a victim – a victim of life, of war, of medicine. She started to feel that she had wasted her life. She told Lise: "I sometimes feel sick in my stomach with the whole situation. I just cannot sit and do nothing. If I cannot work, I feel so helpless." Little by little, she began to sink to a deep depression. She was losing the will to live.

Whenever Piero saw her so discouraged, he scolded her soundly. "Just think of all the work you have done here," he would say. "Think of how many lives you have saved. Think of how many people you have helped. Do you call this wasting your life?" He reminded her how important she was to him, how important she was to her patients and to the hospital. This was the comfort she needed. She was bolstered by his love and by his concern. She was determined to keep living as long as she could.

When Dominique joined them for Christmas, her presence brought both Lucille and Piero much joy. This was the first Christmas they had spent together in three years and they celebrated quietly at home, happy to be together as a family after what Lucille called "our most turbulent year yet."

∽

The anxiety surrounding the hospital continued into the next year. Another group of rebels, who called themselves the Holy Spirit Mobile Forces, had emerged in northern Uganda. They too were intent on waging war against the government forces and used the same sinister means of doing so.. As Lucille explained in a letter to her sisters: "This is a group of fanatic rebels… They are pseudo religious and they attack people, accuse them of collaborating with the regular army, and often shoot them. Yesterday, we received a wounded man who had managed to escape. He had a serious injury on his arm, a deep gash in the bone at the nape of his neck and signs that he had been strangled."

The rebels also resorted to other more familiar tactics. One group threatened to attack the hospital if they did not hand over a large supply of medicines, sugar, salt, and soap. (Piero gave them the salt and soap but not the drugs). Another scaled the walls of the hospital, tied up the nurses on duty and raided the pharmacy. They found nothing there because Piero had locked up all the drugs with the army in Gulu.

Most frightening of all was when a gang of the same rebels forced their way into the Sacred Heart Secondary School just six hundred metres from the hospital. They broke into the two student dormitories, gathered up as many young women as they could, pushed them out of the doorway, and led them away into the bush. School officials calculated that the gang of rebels had abducted eighty-eight women. The captives were held for several days before they were released.

As the year progressed, the same rebels resorted to a new weapon: land mines. Planted along the roads, land mines caused horrendous human damage. The rebels also subjected people to unspeakable forms of torture. For weeks on end, the wounded would stagger into the hospital with cut lips, amputated limbs, and severed genitals. "These gangs are wounding people in ways that are indescribable," Lucille told Lise, and her temper soared as she wrote. "In almost twenty years of war, I thought I had seen everything but even I am shocked by such injuries. They are raping women, and they are kidnapping children to sell as slaves to the Sudanese or to turn them into guerrilla fighters for their own armies. It is all too terrible."

Hundreds of people suffered from these savage acts. "There is not one single family which has not had a parent or a child killed, beaten, kidnapped, or raped," she added. "I can assure you that life for them has become almost unbearable."

⚭

Lucille had great difficulty coming to grips with this new and barbarous type of warfare. She shared her thoughts in another letter to her sister: "I cannot imagine how anyone can treat others in such a dreadful way.

It is truly despicable." She felt sad and depressed and wondered when things would ever change. She had also received news that her father had died, which made her sink even deeper into despair.

Things began to seem so hopeless that Piero, too, started to feel discouraged and dejected. On 14 February 1989, he wrote to his brother Corrado:

"How can you live for three years among all this misery and violence? How can you continue to keep fighting against all these difficulties? How can you not feel that everything you have done amounts to nothing?… We are losing hope and without hope, life is no longer life… We have never been so close to abandoning everything here."

Lucille's health was a growing concern to Piero. She continued to lose weight and felt more and more tired. But, in spite of her disease and the fact that she was now sixty years old, she still managed to do several of the more complicated operations each week. More than ever, her work was important to her. She saw each operation as a challenge, a chance to save a life.

Such was the case with a little boy whose mother brought him into the hospital suffering from an enlarged colon. This malformation could lead to the child's death and would require a delicate operation. Lucille was the only one who could do it. The operation took her four hours to complete. She was exhausted when she finished, but when she saw that the child was going to live, her spirits were enormously boosted.

∞

Many of the staff members were nervous and on edge. They were all deeply affected by the ever-growing presence of AIDS around them. Some had family members who had succumbed to the disease, and each day they saw more and more AIDS patients arrive at the hospital to seek help. Every second patient in the tuberculosis wing now had AIDS; gradually the staff turned the wing into an AIDS unit.

The onset of AIDS created new challenges for the hospital staff. All their working lives they had dedicated themselves to curing patients. Now, they had to resign themselves to treating the patients as best they could. They had to face a heart-breaking reality: there was no cure for AIDS.

The disease had also produced a new and unexpected phenomenon. Pregnant women who had AIDS were dying soon after giving birth, and the hospital was being left with many motherless babies who carried the virus. (Babies born to a mother with AIDS have a 40 per cent chance of carrying the disease.) Normally, family members cared for orphaned children. As the disease began to spread and many family members were also stricken, the babies with AIDS were now being abandoned. Lacor Hospital rallied by setting up an orphanage on the grounds to provide a home for these unwanted babies.

Although Uganda was quick to attack the AIDS epidemic, the number of cases rose dramatically. More than fifteen thousand people, in a population of around eighteen million, had contracted the disease by the end of the 1980s. And the figures would continue to rise.

꩜

Lucille was still examining outpatients every morning. An increasing number of these showed the symptoms of AIDS. As she diagnosed one case after another, she found herself wondering: *How long could I have been carrying the virus?*

She knew it was impossible to have proof exactly when she was contaminated, but it was certainly before the virus was discovered and before the danger of contact with contaminated blood was known. One evening in 1989 when she and Piero were relaxing in their home, they tried to speculate how and when she contracted the disease. Lucille thought it was most likely during her war surgery in 1979, when she performed over one thousand operations for gunshot wounds during the "war of liberation." Piero agreed. "So you see," Lucille concluded with a sigh of resignation, "I have probably been carrying the virus for ten years."

In many ways, Lucille had been lucky. HIV had been identified in 1983, and she was able at least to know the cause of her many illnesses. She was lucky to have access to drugs that helped delay the progression of the disease, and she was under the care of an exceptional doctor, Anthony Pinching.

But most of all, she was bolstered by the love and support of Piero and his family, of her own family in Canada, and of her daughter Dominique. Lucille considered herself to be fortunate that she was not alone in her ongoing battle.

11

Remission

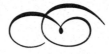

I haven't felt so well in a long time... Once
again, I am working a lot, about ten hours a day,
with enthusiasm and passion. We now have six
Ugandan interns and five Ugandan doctors so at
last, Piero and I, and the three Italian sisters, are
the only white faces in the hospital.
 – Lucille Teasdale, 26 October 1991

As her health slowly deteriorated, Lucille recognized
that she needed to conserve her energy more carefully. She realized too that she required more rest than
before. After all, she had already lived twice as long as the
two years that Anthony Pinching had predicated in 1985.
With any luck, she could defeat the odds even further.

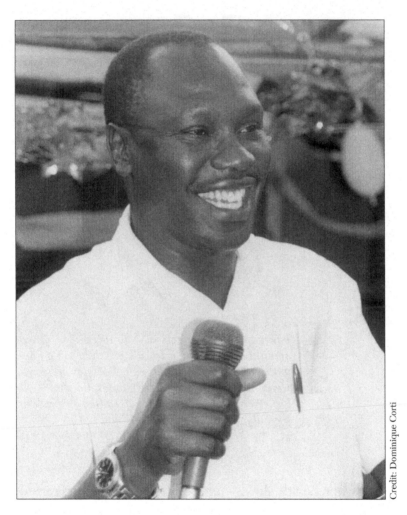

Matthew Lukwiya. Lucille and Piero saw this bright young doctor as a possible successor. He was one of the first Ugandan doctors to carry out his internship at Lacor Hospital.

In March 1989, she and Piero decided to take a short holiday in Kenya over the Easter weekend. They left the hospital in the hands of their trusted lieutenant, Matthew Lukwiya, who was both a gentle and compassionate person and an excellent doctor and administrator. They felt totally confident leaving him in charge while they were away.

They set out from the hospital early on Good Friday morning. They were well on their way to Kampala when a gang of fifty armed rebels, another group belonging to the Holy Spirit Mobile Forces, burst into the hospital grounds. Waving spears and arrows, machetes, and grenades, the rebels demanded to speak to "the Doctor."

"Doctor Corti is not here," explained the guard.

"Give us Dr. Lucille then," they shouted.

"She is not here either," said the guard.

By this time, Matthew had been woken by the loud voices; he dressed and ran to the gate. "Hand over all the drugs," the rebels demanded.

"There are no drugs kept in the compound," Matthew explained.

"We do not believe you," said their leader. "You are refusing our request? Then we will kidnap some of the nuns so we can exchange them for drugs."

Matthew was dumbfounded. He could not believe what he was hearing. He said in a calm voice: "Do you realize that the nuns are very old women who have done a great deal for your own families?" His voice broke as he added. "For many years, these women have cared for your mothers and your sisters."

"Enough," shouted the boss, who was clearly impatient. In the same gruff tone, he ordered the rebels to march over to the residence and seize the nuns.

Matthew jumped in their path. "No, no," he begged. "Don't take the nuns. Take me instead."

They paused for a split second, and then replied. "Fine, but you are only one. So we will take you and some of the nurses as well."

In a flash, they gathered six of the nurses, and Matthew found himself being led with them out of the compound. The rebels marched the group across the countryside. They followed a stream that wound through several banana plantations until they reached their destination.

By this time, Lucille and Piero were dining in the Kenyan seaport of Mombasa. Half way through the meal, a waiter brought them an urgent phone message informing them of the kidnapping. They were shaken by the news and decided at once that, for the safety of the staff and patients, they must close the whole hospital and admit only cases of the utmost emergency.

The couple returned immediately to Lacor and found that the remaining doctors had already left for Kampala, most of the nurses had gone home, and all the nursing students had been transferred to Gulu to finish their courses. Of the patients, only about forty serious cases remained, mostly children.

Lucille and Piero and the few remaining staff members cared for them. Should the couple have needed to find a reason for remaining at Lacor during that time of terror and upheaval, they would have found it in those children. Thanks to the two doctors' loving care, all their young patients survived.

Late one night, the hospital guard knocked on Lucille and Piero's door. Piero opened it to find the guard grinning from ear to ear. Behind him stood a tired and bedraggled Matthew. Lucille shrieked with joy and hugged him like her own child. Everyone was relieved to have Matthew safely home again. His spirits were high although he was weak and thin and suffering from a bout of malaria. He and the nurses had been held hostage for seven days.

The next day, all the nurses were returned. Matthew said their release had been made possible by another group of rebels, former officers of Idi Amin. They had once been treated at Lacor Hospital, they said, and they had never forgotten the good care they had received.

⁓

By now, the hospital was almost deserted. Only a handful of devoted staff members remained – Sister Lina, Brother Elio, half a dozen Ugandan nurses, and of course, Lucille and Piero. They kept themselves cloistered inside one of the buildings, for they all felt it was too unsafe to go outside. Meanwhile, Piero circulated a leaflet to all the local authorities. It read: "The hospital will reopen only when the security of the patients and the staff is assured… Because of the war, thousands of children are dying of measles, of malnutrition and from lack of medical care… Only peace will allow them to stop dying."

Lucille still managed to do a few emergency operations each day. "We are virtually closed except for 'life-threatening emergencies' that cannot be treated by the hospital in Gulu," she wrote to her sister. "All the doctors have left, so we are the only two, exactly like the day when we arrived twenty-eight years ago. There are still the wonderful Italian sisters, of whom two are now eighty years old, and twenty-four nurses.

"I still do a few operations each day. Yesterday, I did three Caesareans. I also operated on a child of four with a blocked intestine and another patient with cancer of the uterus. That one took me three hours to finish and I was exhausted by the end…"

When she wasn't working, Lucille would spend her time at home, reading and listening to her favourite records in an effort to calm her fears. She had never felt so alone. "We feel so isolated and abandoned by God and by man," she told Lise. She opened a leather-bound diary she had begun to keep and, on 17 May 1989, she wrote in large capital letters: I AM VERY FRIGHTENED.

The hospital remained closed for almost six weeks. The tension eased a little after Piero had learned that the rebels' front line had moved farther west. Thanks to strong pressure from many friends of the hospital – forcefully lead by Lucille and Piero – the authorities finally agreed to provide a thirty-man militia to patrol the boundaries of the compound. With this assurance, the hospital reopened.

The Ugandan doctors, including the indispensable Matthew, returned. As word spread, a trickle of patients began to arrive at the gates. Soon, the trickle became a flood and work began to escalate once again.

No one was happier than Lucille, who set to work with renewed energy. Her work made her feel useful, and she found even greater satisfaction from it than she had before. As more and more patients arrived at her door, she was happy to care for them and to help to restore them to health. Without knowing it, her patients were also helping to restore Lucille's sagging spirits.

∞

Piero had managed to recruit several excellent Ugandan interns to help Lucille, especially in the operating theatre. She would hand over to them some of the simpler operations and supervise from the sidelines. For the more difficult operations, she would perform the essential part of the procedure while the interns watched; then they would continue under her supervision.

During one of her high moments, she wrote to Lise: "I am still working a lot, about ten hours a day, with enthusiasm and passion. This week I did several very important and difficult operations... We now have six Ugandan interns and five Ugandan doctors, so Piero and I, and the three Italian sisters, are the only white faces in the hospital. That has always been our dream."

In spite of Lucille's renewed enthusiasm for her work, she still tired easily. She took cortisone regularly to alleviate the incessant bouts of fever. She saw this as a period of remission that allowed her, for the time being at least, to forget her disease and plan a trip to Japan.

The couple had been invited by the Sasakawa Foundation, the organization that had honoured them in 1986, to deliver a speech at a major conference in Tokyo. They left Matthew in charge and on 27 May 1989 set out with Dominique for Tokyo.

Visiting Japan was a dream come true for Lucille. Never before had she spoken to such a large audience, and she was quivering with nervousness as she mounted the podium. But the audience was enthralled by her message and gave her a standing ovation. The following day, she and Piero toured the city. They strolled wide-eyed through the Ginza, Tokyo's fashionable shopping district, and walked along laneways lined with pink cherry blossoms. They visited temples and palaces and squatted on floor mats to sample trays full of sushi. Lucille kept thinking, *This is all such a contrast to Gulu!*

On their return to Lacor, they were relieved to find that there was relative peace in the region and the number of patients at the hospital had more than quadrupled in their absence. There were now four hundred patients for only three hundred beds!

There was another surprise in store for Lucille. During their absence, Piero had arranged for the completion of a new TB wing with ninety beds, which brought the total number of hospital beds to 450. The minute they arrived back home, Piero led Lucille over to see the facility. They walked through the new wing with great excitement. "And now," said Piero, steering Lucille to one end of the new building, "here is a special treat for you!" With a dramatic flourish, he threw open the door to reveal a sparkling new operating theatre! Lucille was almost speechless with joy. That same afternoon, she christened the theatre by performing her first operation in the new facility.

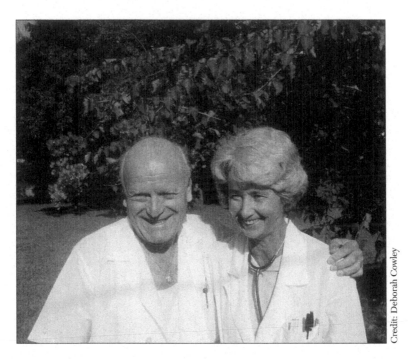

Credit: Deborah Cowley

After thirty-five years of marriage,
Lucille and Piero remained the most devoted of couples.

12

A Will to Survive

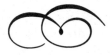

Somehow, after more than ten years with this disease, I always manage to recover. I do not know if it is a miracle, with so many friends and relatives praying for me. Or maybe it is just my stubbornness, or my strong will to survive that is responsible...
– Lucille Teasdale, October 1994.

As the 1990s unfolded, Uganda was showing the first signs of recovery. Security had been greatly improved, the roads were under repair, and electricity had finally been reconnected after four years.

A huge immunization project was starting up again, and the government was taking serious steps to revive the ailing tourism industry. Best of all, there appeared to be relatively strong leadership under President Museveni. At long last, cautious optimism began to spread throughout the country.

Lucille's health continued to fluctuate. She would have low periods, often marked by fever and more weight loss or another bout of shingles. Such setbacks would plunge her into a deep depression for days, sometimes weeks. Then she would bounce back into long and productive days in the operating theatre and with her outpatients. As she explained in a letter to her friend Colette Dion on 29 April 1990: "… I am living on a razor's edge. Between complications, I continue to lead a normal life and to work eight to ten hours a day… For me, the worst thing is the shifting between periods of depression when I am certain that I am finished, that there is nothing to be done and I am about to enter the final stage, and the periods of anxiety when I am convinced that I am becoming just like my mother, a hypochondriac and quite neurotic."

⌒

Lucille and Piero decided to spend a month in Italy to celebrate Christmas with their family. Late one night, they were driving home on a slippery road when suddenly, at a blind intersection, a car smashed into the side of theirs. Piero suffered a cracked rib and Lucille appeared to be unhurt. Later, an X-ray showed that she had fractured her thighbone, but she was able to walk with crutches without too much pain.

After a short recuperation in Italy, they flew back to Uganda, where news of the accident had caused much alarm among the staff. As their car drew up to the hospital gate, a large group of nurses burst into song while a group of excited children jumped up and down, their hands outstretched to greet the couple. "*Safari tye,*" they shouted in Acholi. "Welcome home!"

Lucille stepped out of the car and walked over on her crutches to thank them. From the middle of the crowd, an old woman pushed forward and spoke to her in Acholi. "Dr. Lucille," she said. "Whenever you go away, we are afraid you will never return." She cupped Lucille's hands in hers. "Thank you for coming back to us."

Lucille was deeply touched by the woman's words. *I must keep working as long as I possibly can,* she resolved inwardly.

☙

Lucille and Piero's lifetime work in Uganda now was being recognized outside Africa. They had received many tributes and awards from Italy, but nothing pleased Lucille more than recognition from Canada, the country of her birth. In April 1991, she and Dominique travelled to Ottawa, where Lucille was inducted as a member of the Order of Canada. At a glittering ceremony in Rideau Hall, Governor General Ray Hnatyshyn presented the medal while an aide read a moving citation. "... She has devoted herself to the well-being of the people of northern Uganda for close to thirty years. Together with her pediatrician husband, she has survived through wartorn times to build the hospital into a model training centre and health care facility serving the vast rural area of Gulu."

Soon after, Lucille received another boost – both mentally and physically – with the news that Dominique had become engaged to be married. Her fiancé, Contardo Vergani, was a young surgeon whom she had met at medical school in Milan. Lucille and Piero were thrilled for their daughter. "The news of Dominique's engagement brought us the greatest possible joy," Lucille wrote with excitement to her sister. She and Piero travelled to Milan for the wedding, which took place on 17 November 1993.

Lucille kept on working, sometimes up to ten hours a day, with a compulsion that amazed those around her. She said in an interview, "I wanted to show those living with this disease that you can be well enough to live a happy and full life." But all the time, she was still plagued by different illnesses. She was struck with a bout of tuberculosis and a fifth attack of shingles, which required intravenous treatments three times a day. When the shingles abated, she contracted a severe case of pneumonia. "That one brought me very near to death," she said.

Added to everything else was the sudden appearance of a condition called thrush. Tiny ulcers formed in her mouth and were so painful that Lucille lost most of her appetite and often would not eat for days. The only way to alleviate the pain was to cover her mouth with a purple liquid called gentian violet. "Why don't you paint my whole face with that stuff?" she suggested to Piero. "I think it would be fun to have a purple face!"

She never lost her sense of humour. When a young nurse asked her "What will we do when you die?" Lucille replied, "Don't worry. I will be buried over on that hill with my toes pointing towards the hospital and I will be watching you every single minute!"

In October 1994, Lucille wrote to Lise: "I continue to have highs and lows. My fracture has finally healed and I can now walk without crutches. I can still work with the outpatients five or six hours a day and that pleases me very much. There are times when I don't feel very well... but most of the time, I feel quite calm and serene. Happily, I can still enjoy the simple pleasures of life: a beautiful sunny day, an unexpected letter, a conversation on the radio-telephone with Dominique, or reading a few good books.

"Somehow, after more than ten years with this disease, I always manage to recover. I do not know if it is a miracle, with so many friends and relatives praying to different saints for me. Or maybe it is just my strong will to survive – some would call it stubbornness – that is responsible.

"I do know that every single day, I am happy to be alive. I am happy to be able to enjoy life, to enjoy the love of my husband and my daughter. I do not see why I should live in anguish because I have this disease. When you are a surgeon, it is a risk of the profession."

As Lucille's health deteriorated, her friends and family began to speculate how much longer she could stay in Uganda. When an interviewer put it to her directly, she replied, "Piero cannot live without the hospital. I cannot live without Piero. Now, does that answer your question?"

∞

Many people marvelled at how Lucille managed to continue her struggle for so many years. She attributed it to what she called "moral strength." She told a visiting journalist, "I am very lucky to have been born with this moral strength. You either have it or you don't. If you have it, you can keep on facing all the difficulties that turn up every day. If you do not have it and if you reach that point when you feel you just can't take it any more, then you pack up your suitcase and go back home.

"But if you are convinced by what you are doing, if you truly believe in it, then you stay. There is no other way."

Lucille and Piero could be proud that they had achieved their goal. The tiny forty-bed clinic that they first saw thirty-five years before had become a full medical complex with 450 beds and some of the best facilities in the country. The hospital was serving over 150,000 patients a year, and more importantly, employing over four hundred young medical professionals, all of them Africans who had been trained at Lacor.

Another accolade reached Lucille and Piero in June 1995 in the form of a letter from UN Secretary-General Boutros Boutros-Ghali, who sent Lucille his congratulations and informed her she had received the African Cause Award, official recognition by the United Nations of her work in Africa.

"Your dedicated years of service providing health care to African communities... are an example to us all," the letter read. "Now that you have yourself contracted HIV, and the disease AIDS, your strength of spirit in continuing to work, both as a doctor and as a patient, adds even greater moral authority, and added poignancy, to your life's work. Your courage and commitment in facing this deadly virus, in speaking out boldly about how it has affected you personally, and how it has affected the lives of millions of Africans, are both an example and an inspiration...

"Your sustained work in Uganda is a living testament to the fact that people who contract HIV and AIDS can and do lead full and productive lives. Your tireless advocacy and care for the health and well-being of your patients and your personal commitment to make a difference to the lives of those Africans infected and affected by HIV and AIDS, has left a real and indelible impact. It is my firm conviction that future generations – and many who are alive today – will reap benefits from your work and your example.

"We salute you, and your husband and partner, Dr. Piero Corti, for the tremendous contribution you have made in seeking to help your community in Africa..."

∞

Far from sitting back and resting on their laurels, Lucille and Piero both recognized that it was important to ensure the continuation of the hospital after they were gone. In 1995, they established the Lucille Teasdale and Piero Corti Foundation, and during the last months of her life, Lucille worked tirelessly to raise funds for the Foundation. She travelled with Piero throughout Europe and North America, speaking to governments and non-governmental organizations, to service clubs and church groups. This fundraising was an important challenge, and in spite of her failing health, she met it admirably. When a television interviewer asked her whether it might be time to retire, Lucille shot back: "Why should we retire? To stay at home in a rocking chair? *NO WAY!*"

༎

By the spring of 1996, it became clear that Lucille could no longer remain in Uganda. She was growing weaker, and she knew she did not have long to live. She felt she would be more comfortable in Italy, where she could spend the remainder of her days close to Dominique and to Piero's family. In mid-April, she and Piero left Uganda. Lucille had to say her final farewell to the country she had come to love.

When the time came for Lucille and Piero to leave the hospital, the staff gathered to say goodbye. They hugged her warmly, sang songs, and called out greetings. They knew this was the last time they would see their beloved *Min Atim* – "mother of one born in a foreign land," the name they had given her when Dominique was born. As the car drew away, there was barely a dry eye among them.

The couple flew to Italy and moved into the small house they had rented in Besana, close to Piero's family. Soon after their arrival, Lucille received a message from Canada bringing the news that she had been awarded an honorary doctorate from the Université de

Montréal, the same university where she had received her medical degree forty-one years ago. She was too sick to attend the ceremony, but Lise accepted the award on her behalf and carried the document to Italy to share with Lucille. Lise then stayed on to care for her sister during her last days.

Lucille was now losing strength daily. On 1 August 1996, she sensed that the end was near. Piero sat by her bedside, gently stroking her head. "You know how much I love you, Lucille," he told her, over and over. Dominique stayed close to her mother's side and held her hand while Lise cradled her sister in her arms. Lucille made one final effort to sit up, and then lay back, closed her eyes, and died. She was sixty-seven.

Lucille's coffin was placed in the salon of the house, a crucifix at its foot. Hundreds of people came from all over Italy to pay their respects – family and friends, former medical staff, and many of the Comboni Sisters who had returned to Italy on their retirement.

The priest arrived at the house and led a long procession of mourners who followed the coffin through the rain-swept streets to the church, where they joined in a service of thanksgiving for the life of the woman they had loved and admired.

A few days later, Piero boarded a plane with the coffin of his beloved wife and flew to Uganda. Lucille's body was buried at Lacor among the people she had cared for. Her spirit lives on through the work of those doctors, nurses, and patients she and her husband so inspired.

She will long be remembered as the "doctor of courage."

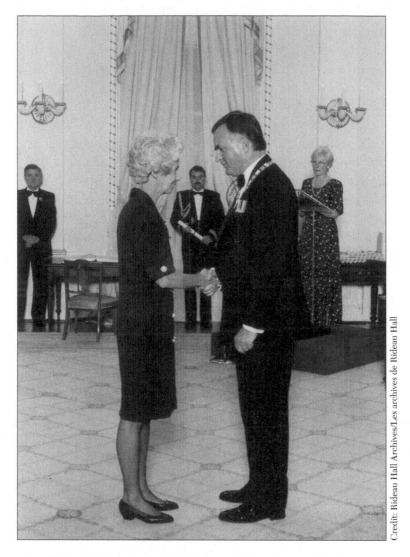

Lucille is presented with the Order of Canada, Canada's highest honour, by Governor General Ray Hnatyshyn.

Epilogue

After Lucille's death in 1996, Lacor Hospital continued to flourish. Piero travelled constantly to raise funds for the Lucille Teasdale and Piero Corti Foundation. Dominique, now a medical doctor and the Foundation's president, along with Lucille's sisters Monique and Lise, carries on the work of the Foundation that Lucille and Piero so ably set in place.

The hospital is now one of the largest and most important medical centres in Uganda. In 2004, thirty-five doctors handled 35,000 admissions and examined over 230,000 outpatients, 60 per cent of them children under six. Two hundred resident students include newly graduated Ugandan doctors serving as interns plus those undergoing training to be nurses, technicians, or nursing assistants. All 550 of the hospital's employees are Ugandans.

The hospital continues to shelter refugees and treat war injuries. It has also become an important research centre for the treatment and prevention of AIDS in Uganda.

AIDS continues to take a heavy human toll in Uganda, but many people are encouraged by the fact that the HIV infection rate has dropped from 14 per cent to less than 8 per cent in the last decade, a direct result of a vigorous national prevention and education program.

∞

Lucille Teasdale's selfless contribution to Uganda has been recognized in many ways:
- A $4.6 million television docudrama, *Dr. Lucille: The Lucille Teasdale Story*, was released in English, French, and Italian in 2000.
- A television documentary film, *In Search of Lucille: The Woman Behind the Surgeon's Mask*, was screened in 2001.
- A television documentary film, *Before I Go: Lucille Teasdale*, was made in 1994.
- A *Historica Minute* on Lucille Teasdale's life has been shown in over 1,000 theatres across Canada.
- A biography of Lucille Teasdale and Piero Corti, *Un rêve pour la vie* by Michel Arseneault, was published in French in 1997.
- A permanent exhibit at the *Canada and the World Pavilion* in Ottawa, Canada, features a panel on the life and work of Lucille Teasdale.
- A commemorative postage stamp was issued in Canada in January 2000 to honour Lucille Teasdale.

CŒ

Dr. Matthew Lukwiya was appointed medical superintendent of Lacor Hospital in 1998. Two years later,
when the highly contagious virus called Ebola swept
through northern Uganda, Matthew Lukwiya was at
the forefront of the battle to contain the outbreak.
There were many casualties among the hospital staff.
One of the last to succumb to the disease was Matthew
himself. He died on 5 December 2000, aged forty-one.

CŒ

Piero Corti carried on working at the hospital and raising funds for the Lucille Teasdale and Piero Corti
Foundation. He died of pancreatic cancer at his home
in Italy on 20 April 2003. Both he and Matthew were
buried next to Dr. Lucille in the shade of the frangipani tree.

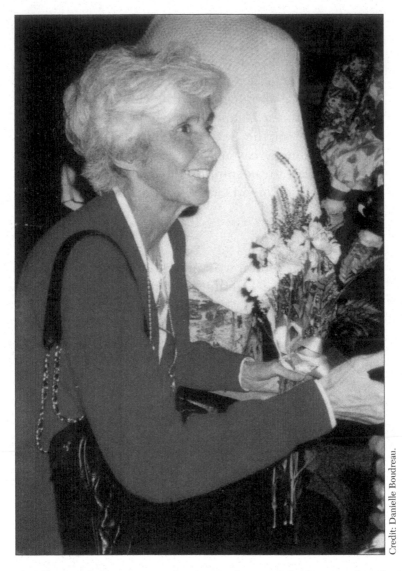

Lucille Teasdale in Montreal in 1995. She spent the last months of her life campaigning tirelessly on behalf of the Foundation she and Piero Corti founded to ensure the future of Lacor Hospital.

Chronology of Lucille Teasdale (1929-1996)

Compiled by Valerie Frith

TEASDALE AND HER TIMES	CANADA AND THE WORLD
	1900
	In East Africa, the Buganda Agreement places the kingdom of Buganda under British administration.
	1921
	In Canada, Mackenzie King is elected Liberal prime minister, a position he will hold until 1948, except for a brief interval in 1926 and during R.B. Bennett's Conservative tenure (1930-1935).
	Agnes Macphail becomes the first woman elected to the Canadian Parliament.
	1923
	Frederick Banting wins the Nobel Prize for discovering insulin.

TEASDALE AND HER TIMES

1925
Piero Corti is born in Besana in Brianza, Italy.

1929
Lucille Teasdale is born in Montreal.

CANADA AND THE WORLD

1925
Tuberculosis (TB) kills 3,000 in Quebec (800 in the Montreal area).

1926
Buganda's British Governor resigns as his administrators demand that the Bugandan chiefs' powers be reduced.

1928
Alexander Fleming discovers penicillin.

1929
The New York Stock Exchange collapses. A ten-year economic crisis begins for the western world.

1930
South African microbiologist Max Theiler develops a yellow-fever vaccine.

1934
Marie Curie, Nobel Prize-winning scientist, dies.

1935
Benito Mussolini, head of Italy's Fascist government, invades Abyssinia (now Ethiopia).

The first sulfa drug is introduced.

1936
Maurice Duplessis and the Union Nationale come to power in Quebec.

TEASDALE AND HER TIMES	CANADA AND THE WORLD
	1937 In Buganda, Asian plantation own-ers are required to give up some property, to provide for small land-holders. Canadian doctor Norman Bethune organizes the Canadian-American Mobile Medical Unit for service in China.
	1939 The Second World War begins, after Germany invades Poland. Canada declares war on Germany and Italy. Norman Bethune cuts himself while operating on a wounded sol-dier and dies, in China, of sep-ticemia (blood poisoning).
	1940 Howard Florey develops penicillin as a practical antibiotic. Women in Quebec are granted the right to vote and to run for office.
1941 Lucille enters the Catholic high school where she will encounter missionary nuns from an orphan-age in China.	**1941** In December, following the Japanese attack on Pearl Harbor, the United States (U.S.) declares war on Japan and its allies, Germany and Italy. Canada declares war on Japan. In the Hyde Park Declaration, Mackenzie King and U.S. Presi-dent Franklin Roosevelt agree to

TEASDALE AND HER TIMES	CANADA AND THE WORLD

permanent joint defence arrangements.

1942
Following a plebiscite, the Canadian Parliament passes Bill 80 in favour of conscription. In Quebec, Maxime Raymond founds the Bloc populaire, a federal party opposed to conscription.

In France, almost half of the Canadian troops who land at Dieppe are killed.

1944
Allied Forces land on the Normandy beaches of France in the D-Day invasion of June 6; the Canadian Army loses 5000 men in the Battle of Normandy.

1945
V-E Day (May 8) marks the Allies' victory in Europe. Germany is divided into four zones.

1947
Britain grants India its independence.

1948
Louis Saint-Laurent succeeds Mackenzie King as Liberal prime minister of Canada.

Mahatma Gandhi is assassinated in India

The World Health Assembly meets for the first time in Geneva.

TEASDALE AND HER TIMES	CANADA AND THE WORLD
	1949 Canada joins the North Atlantic Treaty Organization (NATO). Newfoundland becomes Canada's tenth province. Bugandan rioters burn down the houses of pro-British chiefs. Apartheid is implemented in South Africa.
1950 Lucille enters the medical school at the Université de Montréal. She is one of only eight women in a class of 110.	**1950** Antihistamines become popular remedies for colds and allergies.
1951 Lucille appears on the cover of *Le Petit Journal*'s October edition.	**1951** Nellie McClung, Canada's tireless campaigner for women's rights, dies. In Ottawa, Charlotte Whitton is elected Canada's first female mayor. In the U.S., 400,000 pounds of penicillin and 350,000 pounds of streptomycin are produced.
	1952 A new British governor is appointed to prepare the "larger Uganda framework" for independence. In Kenya, a state of emergency is declared, due to Mau Mau disturbances.

TEASDALE AND HER TIMES	CANADA AND THE WORLD
	Effective drugs that combat TB are introduced.
1953 Piero Corti qualifies as a radiologist.	**1953** Unification of Northern Rhodesia, Southern Rhodesia, and Nyasaland is discussed at the London Conference.
	The King of Buganda is deported for refusing to co-operate with the plan for a united Uganda.
	1954 Dr. Jonas Salk, who has developed a serum against polio, begins inoculating American schoolchildren.
1955 Lucille graduates *cum laude* from medical school. Her internship begins at Ste-Justine's hospital for children.	**1955** The King of Buganda is reinstated.
	Dorothy Hodgkin discovers a treatment for pernicious anemia.
Piero Corti begins three years of training at Ste-Justine's, where he will meet Lucille Teasdale.	
	1956 In Quebec, Maurice Duplessis is re-elected.
	Albert Sabin develops an oral vaccine against polio.
1957 Matthew Lukwiya is born in Uganda.	**1957** John Diefenbaker, a Conservative, is elected prime minister of Canada.

TEASDALE AND HER TIMES	CANADA AND THE WORLD
	Lester B. Pearson receives the Nobel Peace Prize for his role in the Suez Crisis.
1958 Piero leaves Montreal for Africa and India, to visit medical facilities and projects.	**1958** Publicly funded hospitalization insurance is implemented in Canada.
	Ellen Fairclough is the first Canadian woman to serve as a federal cabinet minister.
	Charles de Gaulle is elected president of France.
1959 In Lacor (Uganda), St. Mary's Hospital opens as a dispensary staffed by the Comboni Catholic Missionaries.	**1959** In Canada, The St. Lawrence Seaway opens.
	Severo Ochoa and Arthur Kornberg win a Nobel Prize for synthesizing RNA and DNA.
1960 Lucille completes her surgical training and begins her internship in pediatric surgery in Marseilles, France.	**1960** Jean Lesage's Liberals are elected in Quebec. The Quiet Revolution begins. René Lévesque becomes a member of the Lesage cabinet.
Piero visits Lucille in Marseilles and invites her to join him in Uganda for two or three months.	Milton Obote founds the Uganda People's Congress. The Democratic Party is formed to represent the interests of Catholics.
Lucille spends Christmas in Italy with Piero and his family. She agrees to join him for "a month or two" in Uganda.	The Kenya Constitutional Conference opens to a boycott by African delegates.
	Nigeria becomes independent.

TEASDALE AND HER TIMES

CANADA AND THE WORLD

At Sharpeville, in South Africa, sixty-seven protesters against apartheid are shot by police.

John F. Kennedy becomes president of the U.S.

F.M. Burnet and P.B. Medawar receive a Nobel Prize for discovering acquired immunity against foreign tissue.

1961
In May, Piero and Lucille arrive at St. Mary's in Lacor. Lucille will be the hospital's only surgeon.

After four months, Lucille decides to return to France to complete her course. Piero urges her to return and to marry him. Lucille postpones her decision.

As a result of Piero's fundraising efforts, four cargo planes arrive in Uganda with ten tonnes of equipment for the hospital.

Lucille agrees to marry Piero and to return to Lacor. She visits his family in Italy and her own in Montreal.

Lucille and Piero marry on 4 December, in the chapel at St. Mary's Hospital.

1961
The New Democratic Party of Canada is formed, with T.C. Douglas as its leader.

The United Nations (UN) General Assembly condemns apartheid. South Africa declares its intention to leave the Commonwealth.

The Tanganyika Conference discusses measures to protect African wildlife.

UN Secretary-General Dag Hammarskjöld dies in an air crash while he is in Africa to deal with a crisis in the Congo.

In the U.S., Freedom Riders campaigning against racial segregation are attacked by white citizens.

The U.S. enters the Vietnam War by sending in military advisers.

The Berlin Wall, dividing East from West, is constructed in East Germany.

TEASDALE AND HER TIMES

1962
St. Mary's Hospital is renamed St. Mary's-Lacor. Soon, it will be known simply as Lacor Hospital. Lucille takes charge of a three-month training program for Italian student doctors.

Interns from Makerere University in Kampala begin to come to Lacor for surgical training.

In November, a daughter, Dominique, is born to Lucille and Piero.

CANADA AND THE WORLD

1962
Tanganyika and Uganda become independent. Milton Obote, a northerner, is the first prime minister of Uganda.

In Britain, the Commonwealth Immigration Bill abolishes the principle of an open door to all Commonwealth citizens.

The Cuban Missile Crisis brings the U.S. and the U.S.S.R. to the brink of nuclear war.

F.H. Crick, M.H.F. Wilkins, and J.D. Watson share a Nobel Prize for determining the molecular structure of DNA.

The morning-sickness drug, Thalidomide, is shown to produce birth defects.

1963
Liberal Lester B. Pearson is elected prime minister of Canada.

Kenya becomes independent.

U.S. President John F. Kennedy is assassinated in Dallas, Texas.

1964
In Uganda, Idi Amin becomes Prime Minister Obote's right-hand man in the military, where he is rapidly promoted.

TEASDALE AND HER TIMES	CANADA AND THE WORLD
	Units of the Ugandan army mutiny. British troops are called in to restore order.

1965
Canada's Maple Leaf flag replaces the Red Ensign, symbol of the British Empire.

In Alabama, Martin Luther King leads a march for the rights of black Americans.

1966
The Union Nationale, under Daniel Johnson, is elected in Quebec.

Britain bans all trade with Rhodesia (now Zimbabwe).

The Bechuanaland protectorate becomes the republic of Botswana.

In China, Chairman Mao launches the People's Cultural Revolution.

1967
In Quebec, René Lévesque resigns from the Liberal Party and founds le Mouvement souveraineté-association (Sovereignty-Association Movement).

Expo 67, the world's fair, is held in Montreal as Canada celebrates the 100th birthday of Confederation.

French President Charles de Gaulle exhorts a Montreal crowd, *"Vive le Québec! Vive le Québec libre!"*

TEASDALE AND HER TIMES	CANADA AND THE WORLD

The new Ugandan constitution abolishes the traditional kingdoms.

The East African Community is formed by Kenya, Tanzania, and Uganda.

1968
At age six, Dominique begins attending the school in Gulu, where her lessons in the early grades are in the Acholi language.

1968
Liberal Pierre Elliott Trudeau is elected prime minister of Canada.

René Lévesque founds the Parti Québécois (PQ) and becomes its first leader.

In the U.S., civil rights leader Martin Luther King is assassinated.

To counter an influx of Kenyan Asians, Britain's Commonwealth Immigration Act is amended.

1969
A three-year civil war begins in the Sudan.

American astronaut Neil Armstrong is the first man to walk on the moon.

1970
In Canada, medicare (universal health insurance) is implemented.

During the October Crisis, British diplomat James Cross and Minister of Labour Pierre Laporte are kidnapped by the Front de la Libération du Québec. Laporte is murdered. The government of

TEASDALE AND HER TIMES	CANADA AND THE WORLD
	Canada invokes the War Measures Act.
	White Rhodesians proclaim an independent republic.
1971 Lucille and Piero send Dominique to school in Italy, for her own safety. She is homesick and unhappy.	**1971** Milton Obote is overthrown in a coup. Idi Amin becomes president of Uganda.
	At the Victoria Conference, Quebec rejects the federal government's proposal to patriate and amend Canada's Constitution.
1972 Lucille and Piero receive the Missione del Medico – Angelo De Gasperis.	**1972** Pierre Elliott Trudeau is re-elected prime minister of Canada, with a minority government.
Dominique leaves Italy to enrol in a Nairobi boarding school. She is now able to return home to Gulu every three months.	In Uganda, Idi Amin expels 70,000 Asians along with all others who insist on retaining their British citizenship. He also nationalizes thirty-four British farms and ten tea estates.
	A 2.5-million-year-old human skull is discovered in northern Kenya.
1973 Lucille and Piero open the Lacor Nursing Training School, with a residence for student nurses.	**1973** North Vietnam and the U.S. sign a ceasefire agreement in Paris.
1974 Matthew Lukwiya completes his Certificate of Education as the top student in northern Uganda.	**1974** In the Canadian federal election, Trudeau's Liberals win a majority government.

TEASDALE AND HER TIMES

CANADA AND THE WORLD

The PQ convention agrees to a referendum strategy for achieving Quebec independence.

1976
The first twenty-five nurses graduate from the Lacor Nursing Training School. The hospital has grown to a 205-bed hospital with two dispensaries, a laboratory, and a radiology department.

Idi Amin visits Lacor Hospital.

Lucille's mother dies in Montreal.

Matthew Lukwiya is Uganda's top student in the Advanced Certificate of Education.

1977
Matthew Lukwiya begins his six years' training at Makerere University Medical School.

1976
René Lévesque becomes premier of Quebec when the PQ wins the provincial election.

The world's first Ebola outbreak is reported in the Sudan. A second outbreak follows in Zaire (now the DR Congo).

A viral cause for multiple sclerosis is discovered.

The first reports on damage to the earth's ozone layer are released.

1977
The East African Community disbands.

Smallpox is declared eradicated, worldwide.

1978
A new human retrovirus is isolated, in a Los Angeles man. (A retrovirus borrows genes from cells and modifies them.)

1979
Lacor Hospital is repeatedly ransacked by the remnants of Idi Amin's disbanded army. Piero suffers a punctured eardrum during one confrontation with marauders.

1979
Joe Clark, a Conservative, becomes prime minister of Canada but remains in power for for less than one year.

Idi Amin is ousted. A Uganda National Liberation Army (UNLA)

TEASDALE AND HER TIMES	CANADA AND THE WORLD

Lacor Hospital closes down its three peripheral community health centres for safety reasons.

By Christmas, a measure of stability has been restored. In the coming year, Lucille and Piero plan to reopen the satellite health centres and to build a new ward for cancer and TB patients.

government is formed; it lasts only sixty-eight days.

A volatile coalition governs Uganda until December 1980.

1980
Trudeau's Liberals are returned to power in Canada.

The first Quebec referendum on sovereignty-association results in a "no" victory.

Milton Obote is returned as president of Uganda. Civil war breaks out.

1981
The PQ is re-elected in Quebec.

The federal government patriates the Canadian Constitution without the consent of Quebec.

The National Resistance Army (NRA) is founded in Uganda.

The Centers for Disease Control (CDC), in Atlanta, Georgia, publish their first two reports on the new human retrovirus.

1982
Victims of a mysterious disease (soon to be known as HIV/AIDS) begin to appear at Lacor Hospital.

1982
At the CDC, the new human retrovirus is named acquired

TEASDALE AND HER TIMES	CANADA AND THE WORLD

Lacor is certified as a teaching hospital.

immune deficiency syndrome (AIDS).

Lucille and Piero receive the Ufficiale al Merito della Repubblica Italiana Award from the President of Italy.

An outbreak of AIDS is reported in the village of Kasensero, Uganda.

1983
Matthew Lukwiya begins his internship at Lacor. He also studies hospital administration in Italy for three months.

1983
Conflict between Uganda and southern Sudan escalates.

1984
Matthew Lukwiya is appointed a medical officer at Lacor Hospital.

1984
Brian Mulroney, a Conservative, is elected prime minister of Canada.

Dominique enrols in the University of Milan's Faculty of Medicine.

Bob Geldorf organizes Band-Aid, for famine relief in Ethiopia.

1985
Lucille learns that she has tested positive for HIV. She concludes that she contracted the disease from wounded soldiers' bone fragments that punctured her surgical gloves.

1985
René Lévesque resigns as Quebec's premier and as leader of the PQ.

Robert Bourassa's Liberals win Quebec's provincial election.

Dr. Anthony Pinching, a specialist in HIV/AIDS, estimates that Lucille has a 25 per cent chance of living for two years. Her surgical activities must be curtailed.

In Uganda, Milton Obote is ousted again. A weak coalition governs until the end of the year, but the NRA is effectively in control of southwestern and northwestern Uganda.

AIDS reaches Kampala.

The first annual international conference on AIDS convenes in

TEASDALE AND HER TIMES	CANADA AND THE WORLD

CANADA AND THE WORLD column:

Atlanta, Georgia. The number of cases reported to the World Health Organization (WHO) has more than doubled within the year.

At the Commonwealth Prime Ministers Conference, Britain's Margaret Thatcher opposes sanctions against South Africa.

1986

1986

The World Health Organization (WHO) awards the Sasakawa Prize to Lucille Teasdale and Piero Corti.

Lucille receives the Paul Harris Award from Rotary International.

Lacor Hospital is caught between the National Resistance Army and the Uganda People's Democratic Army. Staff members begin to flee.

The National Resistance Movement (NRM, formerly the NRA), under President Y.K. Museveni, takes over Uganda's government.

Civil war breaks out again in Uganda, with the NRM and the Uganda National Liberation Army as the main rival factions.

Alice Lakwena, a young Acholi woman, forms the Holy Spirit Mobile Forces (HSMF) in northern Uganda.

The term human immunodeficiency virus (HIV) is introduced, to describe the first stages of AIDS.

1987

Matthew Lukwiya goes to London for three months to study tropical diseases.

In March, Amooti Mwazi, a nurse at Lacor, is abducted by armed rebels. Piero closes the peripheral health centres, as well as the entire

1987

In Canada, René Lévesque dies.

The federal government and the ten provincial premiers sign the Meech Lake Accord.

The number of AIDS cases reported to the WHO has almost

TEASDALE AND HER TIMES	CANADA AND THE WORLD

hospital (except for emergency cases).

doubled (to 96,500) from the previous year.

Amooti Mwazi is released, but she has been tortured. Panic spreads among the Lacor Hospital staff.

The General Assembly of the United Nations (UN) holds its first debate on AIDS.

Hundreds of refugees from Rwanda and the Sudan flock to Lacor Hospital for sanctuary.

The Lord's Resistance Army (LRA) emerges, a new faction in Uganda's civil war.

Lucille receives the Frederick Newton Gisborn Starr Award from the Canadian Medical Association.

The village of Kasensero in Uganda is reported as depopulated by AIDS, five years after its initial outbreak there.

Twice Lucille is forced to fly to London for treatment of injuries complicated by her having AIDS.

Dominique joins her parents for their first Christmas together in three years.

1988
Rebels belonging to the HSMF threaten the hospital and cause widespread suffering in the surrounding region.

1988
The WHO records 145,000 new cases of AIDS but cautions that this is only a fraction of the real total.

Lucille's father dies in Montreal.

Canada signs a commercial free trade agreement with the U.S.

Piero begins to serve as advisor on medical training for Italy's Ministry of External Affairs.

1989
The Lacor Hospital's TB wing is reassigned to AIDS sufferers. An orphanage is established for infants whose mothers have died of the disease.

1989
Bourassa's Liberals are re-elected in Quebec.

General elections are held in Uganda. A moratorium on

TEASDALE AND HER TIMES	CANADA AND THE WORLD

In March, rebels from a a brigade of the HSMF abduct Matthew Lukwiya and six nurses. A week later they are released. But Piero and Lucille declare the hospital closed (except for emergency cases) until the government guarantees their security.

After six weeks, the hospital reopens. A militia force of thirty patrols outside the compound.

Lucille and Piero travel to Japan to speak at a Sasakawa Foundation conference. Dominique accompanies them.

Lacor Hospital's new ninety-bed TB wing opens.

In October, Deborah Cowley visits Lucille Teasdale in Uganda and is the first western journalist to interview her. The following year *Reader's Digest* publishes Cowley's article, "The Hospital of Hope."

1990

With five Ugandan doctors and six interns, Lacor Hospital approaches Lucille and Piero's dream of an all-African staff.

Matthew Lukwiya leaves for a one-year course at the Liverpool Institute of Tropical Hygiene. He receives his master's degree in Tropical Pediatrics, the top student in his class. He declines a lectureship there and returns to

violence is declared in the Gulu district.

The Fifth International Conference on AIDS convenes in Montreal.

The Berlin Wall falls.

1990

In Canada, the Meech Lake Accord dies when Manitoba and Newfoundland refuse to ratify it.

The Bloc Québécois, a federal party with sovereigntist goals, is founded.

The United Democratic Christian Movement (UDCM, formerly the HSMF) mounts new operations in the Gulu region of Uganda.

Teasdale and Her Times	**Canada and the World**
Lacor, where he is put in charge of the pediatric ward.	Germany is reunified.
While in Italy for Christmas, Lucille fractures a thighbone but is soon able to walk on crutches.	
Lucille is recognized by the International Medical Women's Association for her work with AIDS patients.	
1991 Lucille is awarded the Order of Canada.	**1991** Kampala's AIDS Information Centre (AIC) opens, the first clinic of its kind in sub-Saharan Africa.
	1992 In a national referendum, six Canadian provinces (including Quebec) reject the Charlottetown Accord, a proposed constitutional amendment that federal and provincial leaders had agreed to.
	Peace talks begin between the Ugandan government and the LRA.
1993 Dominique Corti marries an Italian surgeon, Contardo Vergani.	**1993** Kim Campbell replaces Brian Mulroney as leader of the Conservative Party. She is the first woman to serve as prime minister of Canada. But in the federal election, Jean Chrétien and the Liberals receive a resounding majority.

Lucille Teasdale

TEASDALE AND HER TIMES

1994

Lacor employs 400 medical professionals, all Africans trained at the hospital, now a 450-bed facility serving 150,000 patients a year.

Lucille receives the Professionalità e Lavoro award for her professionalism and work from the Alliance of Municipalities of Italy.

1995

The UN awards Lucille the African Cause prize.

Lucille and Piero are named Honorary Consultants for the Ugandan Ministry of Health.

Lucille is widely honoured in her home province, Quebec. She receives the Velan Award from the Rotary Club of Montreal, is made a Grand Officier de l'Ordre national du Québec, is cited as a Personalité de l'Année by *La Presse*, is one of Les Grands de l'Année in *L'Actualité* and is voted Femme de l'Année by Radio-Québec's audience.

The Royal College of Physicians and Surgeons of Canada awards Lucille an Honorary Fellowship.

CANADA AND THE WORLD

1994

The PQ, led by Jacques Parizeau, is elected in Quebec.

The Ugandan government and the LRA agree to a ceasefire. Rallies are organized to explain the peace process to the public.

An estimated 800,000 Tutsis and moderate Hutus are killed in 100 days of genocide in Rwanda.

In South Africa, Nelson Mandela becomes the country's first black president.

1995

In Canada, a second Quebec referendum ends with a narrow rejection of sovereignty.

The federal government passes a motion to recognize Quebec as a distinct society.

Christine Silverberg, of Calgary, becomes the first female police chief appointed for a major Canadian city.

Alexa McDonough becomes the leader of the NDP.

Canada's Krever Commission, investigating the "tainted blood" scandal, ends its public hearings with 300 allegations of misconduct against the Red Cross and other agencies.

158

TEASDALE AND HER TIMES	CANADA AND THE WORLD

Lucille and Piero receive Italy's Premio della Professionalità.

Another Ebola outbreak is reported in Zaire.

Lacor Hospital receives the Premio Antonio Feltrinellli for Exceptional Accomplishment of High Moral and Humanitarian Value.

At the Commonwealth Conference, Nigeria is suspended (for abuses of human rights), and Mozambique is admitted, the first member that was never a British colony.

The Lucille Teasdale and Piero Corti Foundation is established.

A ten-year study of Lacor Hospital's activities, co-sponsored by Italy's Istituto Superiore di Sanità, is launched.

1996
Lucille leaves Lacor Hospital and Uganda for the last time.

1996
PQ leader Lucien Bouchard becomes premier of Quebec.

Lucille is awarded an honorary doctorate by the Université de Montréal. Her sister Lise accepts on her behalf.

Heritage Minister Sheila Copps opens the Canadian Information Office, a new agency to promote national unity.

On August 1, Lucille Teasdale dies, in Italy, of AIDS.

More than 15,000 people meet in Vancouver for the eleventh international conference on HIV/AIDS. Significant improvements in treatment are reported.

Lucille Teasdale is buried on the grounds of Lacor Hospital.

People from the villages (especially women and children) begin coming to Lacor Hospital to spend the night safe from looting guerrillas, who kidnap and enslave children or turn them into fighters.

Six UN agencies combine forces and establish UNAIDS, the Joint United Nations Program on HIV/AIDS.

TEASDALE AND HER TIMES	CANADA AND THE WORLD
1997	**1997**
A biography of Lucille Teasdale and Piero Corti, *Un rêve pour la vie* by Quebec journalist Michel Arseneault, is published.	Statistics Canada reports that the wage gap between women and men has narrowed to an average of 73 per cent.
Lacor Hospital sets up a camp inside the hospital compound for internally displaced people. Between 1500 and 2500 people live in the camp, and up to 3000 "night commuters" come to the hospital only for protection during the night.	In the Canadian federal election, the Liberals led by Prime Minister Jean Chrétien are re-elected. The 1982 Constitution Act is amended to allow Quebec to replace its religion-based school system with one drawn along linguistic lines. The plight of thousands of children abducted by the LRA in Uganda receives increasing international attention.
1998	**1998**
Matthew Lukwiya is named medical superintendent of Lacor Hospital. Dominique Corti receives her medical degree from the University of Milan.	The Research Center in New York reports the oldest known case of HIV infection in a sample taken from a man in the Congo, in 1959.
1999	**1999**
The total number of admissions in the pediatric ward at Lacor Hospital has more than doubled over a ten-year period.	Nine of Canada's ten provinces (all but Quebec) sign a Social Accord for implementing social programs. Canadian astronaut Julie Payette takes part in a space shuttle mission.

TEASDALE AND HER TIMES	CANADA AND THE WORLD
	In Ethiopia, a fossil skull reveals a previously unknown species of human ancestor.
2000	**2000**
A docudrama, *Dr. Lucille: The Lucille Teasdale Story*, is released in English, French, and Italian.	Justice Beverley McLachlin is sworn in as the first female Chief Justice of the Supreme Court of Canada.
Matthew Lukwiya receives another master's degree (in Public Health) from Makerere University.	The House of Commons passes the Clarity Bill setting guidelines for the wording of any future Quebec referendum on secession.
Matthew Lukwiya identifies the Ebola virus among patients and nurses at Lacor. He notifies local authorities and the WHO, and he organizes an isolation ward for Ebola patients.	In the federal election, Jean Chrétien's Liberals win a third straight majority.
The Centers for Disease Control install an Ebola laboratory at Lacor Hospital.	Former Prime Minister of Canada Pierre Elliott Trudeau dies on 28 September.
Matthew Lukwiya contracts the Ebola virus and dies of the disease at age 41. He is buried near Lucille Teasdale on the grounds of Lacor Hospital.	In Walkerton, Ontario, a lethal strain of E.coli is discovered in tainted drinking water.
The WHO credits Matthew Lukwiya with limiting the Ebola outbreak to Gulu and two other areas. Besides Lukwiya, twelve more Lacor Hospital staff members are among the Ebola dead.	Uganda and Sudan sign the Winnipeg Communiqué for Immediate Action on Abducted Children.
The American Medical Association names Matthew Lukwiya a Role Model.	

TEASDALE AND HER TIMES	CANADA AND THE WORLD
2001	**2001**
In February, the WHO declares the Ebola outbreak to be over, and full activities resume at Lacor Hospital during April.	Canada's former ambassador to the UN, Stephen Lewis, is named Secretary-General Kofi Annan's Special Envoy for HIV/AIDS in Africa.
2003	**2003**
Piero receives the Paul Harris Award from Rotary International.	Uganda's Ministry of Health reports an outbreak of cholera in the Bundibugyo district.
Piero Corti dies, on Easter Sunday, of pancreatic cancer. He is buried with Lucille Teasdale and Matthew Lukwiya, on the grounds of Lacor Hospital.	Over 20 million people have died since the first cases of AIDS were identified in 1981; UNAIDS estimates that 34-46 million adults and children are living with HIV/AIDS worldwide.
2004	**2004**
In April, Lucille Teasdale and Piero Corti are posthumously awarded the Golden Medal of Civil Valour, the highest award presented by the Republic of Italy for acts of exceptional courage.	After the Canadian federal election, the Liberals, led by Paul Martin, form a minority government.
The number of "night commuters" at Lacor Hospital drops from 10,000 in May to 3000 in October. The high number of refugees within the compound places an enormous strain on the hospital's infrastructure.	The International Criminal Court launches an investigation into crimes against humanity and war crimes in northern Uganda. The court's jurisdiction only extends back to 2002, however.
	In May, the WHO announces an Ebola outbreak in southern Sudan. By August, it is declared over.
	The World AIDS Campaign for 2004 is devoted to "Women, Girls, and HIV/AIDS." In sub-Saharan Africa almost 60 per cent of adults living with HIV are women.

TEASDALE AND HER TIMES

2005
The results of the ten-year study of 155,205 Lacor Hospital patients is published in the *Transactions of the Royal Society of Tropical Medicine and Hygiene*. During 2004 alone, Lacor Hospital's staff of 550 treated 230,000 outpatients and admitted 35,000. The hospital is currently training 200 new medical professionals.

CANADA AND THE WORLD

2005
A polio epidemic unites twenty-two African countries in an immunization campaign.

On 26 December, an earthquake off the west coast of northern Sumatra results in a tsunami that causes widespread devastation and loss of life.

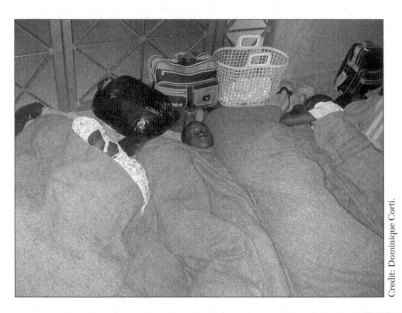

Refugees (especially women and children) come to Lacor Hospital to spend the night safe from guerrillas, who loot the villages and kidnap and enslave children or turn them into fighters.

Acknowledgments

F or this book, I was able to draw on my notes from my visit in 1989 with Lucille and Piero, as well as from a voluminous package of Lucille's letters and papers in the National Archives. I am grateful to archivist Andrée Lavoie, who has meticulously catalogued the papers of Lucille Teasdale and Piero Corti, and whose enthusiasm for my book was encouraging. I owe a great debt to journalist Michel Arseneault, who spent many hours with Lucille and Piero, and whose biography of the couple *Un rêve pour la vie* provided many useful insights. I also appreciate the timely help I received from Sheryl McFarlane and Teresa de Bertodano.

A special bouquet to Don and Elizabeth Hillman, another pair of remarkable doctors, who so generously shared their knowledge of medicine, of Uganda, and of their long-time friends, Lucille and Piero Corti.

Finally, my warm thanks to Lucille Teasdale's sisters Lise and Monique for their assistance and especially to Lucille and Piero's daughter, Dominique Corti, who was unstinting in her support.

The author's proceeds from this book will be donated to:

The Lucille Teasdale & Piero Corti Foundation
Postal Box #206, NDG Branch,
Montreal, Quebec. H4A 3P5
Tel: (514) 237-6054
www.lacorhospital.org

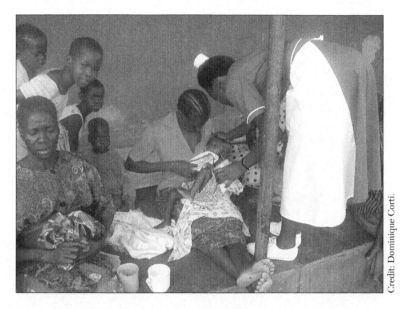

A nurse assists a patient in the courtyard of the hospital.

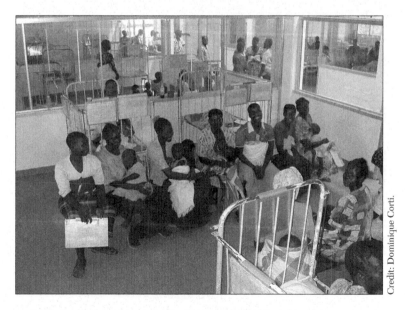

Patients waiting to see the doctor. In 2004, 35,000 patients
were admitted to Lacor Hospital. More than 60 per cent
of these patients were children under six.

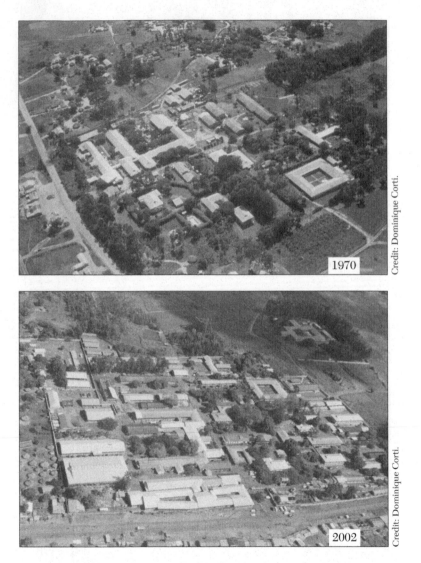

1970

2002

Aerial views showing the expansion of Lacor Hospital
from 1970 to 2002.

Sources Consulted

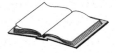

Books

ARSENEAULT, Michel. *Lucille Teasdale et Piero Corti: Un rêve pour la vie.* Montréal (Québec): Éditions Libre Expression, 1997.

KIRSCH, Sharon. *Fabulous Female Physicians. Women's Hall of Fame Series.* Toronto: Second Story Press, 2001.

LAMB, David. *The Africans: Encounters from the Sudan to the Cape.* New York and Toronto: Random House, Inc. and Random House of Canada Limited, 1983.

Articles and Pamphlets

ARSENEAULT, Michel. "A Canadian doctor is paying the ultimate price." *Globe and Mail*, 10 September 1994.

————. "Il est minuit, Dr Teasdale." *L'Actualité*, 15 juin 1994.*

————. "La missionnaire au bistouri." *L'Actualité*, Janvier 1995.*

ATHERTON, Tony. "Canadian missionary doctor inspired Quebec actress." *Ottawa Citizen*, 26 April 2000.

*Written in French

COWLEY, Deborah. "Uganda's Hospital of Hope." *Reader's Digest*, August 1990.

———. "Médecins de l'espoir en Ouganda." *Sélection Reader's Digest*, Août 1990.*

OLOYA, Opiyo. "My hero, the unsung Canadian." *Globe and Mail*, 28 April 2000.

PROULX, Vickie, Bénédicthe Bissonnette-Marcoux, and Marc-André Paquette-Champagne. *Lucille Teasdale*. École secondaire Beaulieu, Février 2003.*

ROBERT, Véronique. "Femme de l'Année: Lucille Teasdale." *Châtelaine*, Janvier 1995.*

"'My God, who is this woman?'" *Ottawa Citizen*, 4 April 2000.

St. Mary's Hospital Story. Tipografia Lucini – Milan. 1961-1981.

Films

Before I go: Lucille Teasdale. Television documentary, produced by Ole Gjerstad and screened on CBC's *Man Alive* in November 1994.

Dr. Lucille: The Lucille Teasdale Story. Television documentary produced by Francine Allaire and starring Marina Orsini. Released April 2000 in French and Italian.

In Search of Lucille: The Woman Behind the Surgeon's Mask. Television documentary by Hélène Klodawsky, produced by Francine Allaire in 2000.

Websites

www.lacorhospital.org (Official website of the Lucille Teasdale and Piero Corti Foundation).

www.histori.ca/minutes/minute.do?ID=10117 (Text of *Historica Minute*, a 60-second "mini-movie" about Lucille Teasdale).

www.virtualmuseum.ca/Exhibitions/Medicentre/en/teas_print.htm (Canadian Medical Hall of Fame)

www.tolerance.ca/GrandesFigures05.asp?Langue=2 ("Lucille Teasdale, Medicine From the Heart," Great Promoters of Tolerance series)

Index

Page numbers in *italics* refer to photographs, maps, or illustrations.

Printed in May 2005
at AGMV/Marquis,
Cap-Saint-Ignace (Québec).